Bacterial and Parasitic Contamination of Blood Components

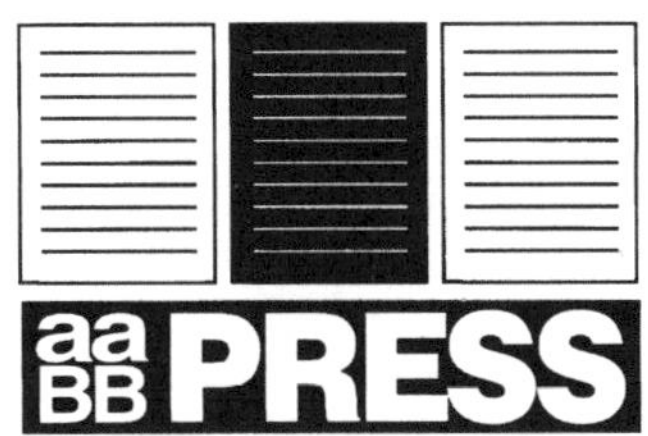

Other related publications from the AABB:

Emerging Technologies in Transfusion Medicine
Edited by Christopher Stowell, MD, PhD, and
Walter H. Dzik, MD

Transfusion Reactions, 2nd Edition
Edited by Mark A. Popovsky, MD

Bacterial and Parasitic Contamination of Blood Components

Editor

Mark E. Brecher, MD
Director, Transplantation and Transfusion Services,
McClendon Clinical Laboratories,
University of North Carolina Hospitals, and
Professor of Pathology and Laboratory Medicine
University of North Carolina at Chapel Hill
Chapel Hill, North Carolina

AABB Press
Bethesda, Maryland
2003

Mention of specific products or equipment by contributors to this AABB Press publication does not represent an endorsement of such products by the AABB Press nor does it necessarily indicate a preference for those products over other similar competitive products.

Efforts are made to have publications of the AABB Press consistent in regard to acceptable practices. However, for several reasons, they may not be. First, as new developments in the practice of blood banking occur, changes may be recommended to the AABB *Standards for Blood Banks and Transfusion Services.* It is not possible, however, to revise each publication at the time such a change is adopted. Thus, it is essential that the most recent edition of the *Standards* be consulted as a reference in regard to current acceptable practices. Second, the views expressed in this publication represent the opinions of authors. The publication of this book does not constitute an endorsement by the AABB Press of any view expressed herein, and the AABB Press expressly disclaims any liability arising from any inaccuracy or misstatement.

The publisher has made every effort to trace the copyright holders for borrowed material. If they have inadvertently overlooked any, they will be pleased to make the necessary arrangements at the first opportunity.

To purchase additional copies of this book, please call our sales department at (301)215-6499 or fax orders to (301)907-6895. AABB sales representatives are available from 8:30 am to 5:00 pm, EST, Monday through Friday, for telephone access. For other book services, including chapter reprints and large quantity sales, ask for the Senior Sales Associate.

Visit the American Association of Blood Banks' Web site on the Internet at www.aabb.org or e-mail our sales department at sales@aabb.org.

American Association of Blood Banks
8101 Glenbrook Road
Bethesda, Maryland 20814-2749

ISBN NO. 1-56395-203-3
Printed in the United States

AABB Press Editorial Board

Contributors

Morris A. Blajchman, MD, FRCP(C)
McMaster University
Canadian Blood Services
Hamilton, Ontario, Canada

Mark E. Brecher, MD
McLendon Clinical Laboratories,
University of North Carolina Hospitals
Chapel Hill, North Carolina

Marla C. Brumit, MD
University of North Carolina Hospitals
Chapel Hill, North Carolina

Ritchard G. Cable, MD
Connecticut Blood Services
Farmington, Connecticut

Mindy Goldman, MD, FRCP(C)
Canadian Blood Services
Ottawa, Ontario, Canada

Shauna N. Hay, MT(ASCP)
University of North Carolina Hospitals
Chapel Hill, North Carolina

Dirk de Korte, PhD
Sanquin Research at CLB
Amsterdam, The Netherlands

Jong-Hoon Lee, MD
Food and Drug Administration
Rockville, Maryland

David A. Leiby, PhD
Jerome H. Holland Laboratory for the Biomedical Sciences
American Red Cross
Rockville, Maryland
George Washington University
Washington, District of Columbia

Sharyn Orton, PhD
Food and Drug Administration
Rockville, Maryland

Louis M. Katz, MD
Mississippi Valley Regional Blood Center
Davenport, Iowa

Elizabeth Palavecino, MD
Citywide Blood Bank Fellowship Program
Cleveland, Ohio

Ira Shulman, MD
University of Southern California Medical Center
Los Angeles, California

Stephen J. Wagner, PhD
American Red Cross Biomedical Research and Development
Rockville, Maryland

Roslyn Yomtovian, MD
University Hospitals of Cleveland
Case Western Reserve University School of Medicine
Cleveland, Ohio

Table of Contents

Preface

PERHAPS ONE OF THE GREAT MEDICAL TRIUMPHS of the late 20th century was the virtual elimination of known viral risk from blood and blood components. With the elimination of viral risk, the residual risk of transfusion-transmitted disease is now predominantly bacterial or parasitic in nature. As we further reduce the risks associated with blood transfusion, with regard to bacteria and parasites, it is important to have a state-of-the-art reference available.

To that end, within this book are gathered chapters by recognized leaders in their fields, covering bacteria, syphilis, malaria, Chagas' disease, and other parasitic infections. In addition to the history, pathology, and epidemiology of these infections, chapters address detection strategies and the potential for pathogen reduction. Particular emphasis is placed on bacterial contamination including avoidance, detection, implementation, and cost-effectiveness. Two association bulletins and a message from the AABB president addressing bacterial contamination appear as appendices to the book, and are provided as a convenience to readers.

I am indebted to the many authors who have made this book possible in a very short time frame and to Shauna Hay for the hours she devoted toward making it a reality. I thank the AABB Press Editorial Board for having the foresight to appreciate the need for such a text.

Mark E. Brecher, MD
Editor

About the Editor

Mark E. Brecher, MD, is director of Transplantation and Transfusion Services at McLendon Clinical Laboratories, University of North Carolina Hospitals, and Professor of Pathology and Laboratory Medicine at the University of North Carolina at Chapel Hill. Dr. Brecher received his medical degree from the University of Chicago in 1982, where he completed a surgical internship and a residency in anatomic/clinical pathology. He received fellowship training in blood bank/ transfusion medicine at the Mayo Clinic and continued as a staff physician with the Mayo Clinic Blood Bank and Transfusion Service from 1988-1992 before relocating to Chapel Hill.

In addition to serving on the editorial boards of *Transfusion* and the *Journal of Clinical Apheresis*, Dr. Brecher is an ad hoc reviewer for several hematology-related periodicals. He has published over 100 articles and many book chapters. He is a two-time editor of both the AABB *Technical Manual* (14th and 15th editions) and *Collected Questions and Answers* (6th and 7th editions).

Dr. Brecher is a member of several professional societies, including the AABB, ASH, ASFA, and AMA. He has served on several AABB committees and spent over a decade as an AABB assessor. He is currently the chair of the DHHS Blood Safety and Availability Committee and remains a popular international lecturer.

Although he maintains an active interest in several areas of transfusion medicine, Dr. Brecher's focus is often on blood conservation, platelet transfusion therapy, mathematical modeling, bacterial contamination, apheresis, and cellular therapy.

Dr. Brecher lives in Chapel Hill with his wife, Maria Brecher, MD, and their two daughters, Danielle and Juliana.

In: Brecher ME, ed.
Bacterial and Parasitic Contamination of Blood Components
Bethesda, MD: AABB Press, 2003

1

Bacterial Contamination of Blood Components—History and Epidemiology

ROSLYN YOMTOVIAN, MD, AND
ELIZABETH PALAVECINO, MD

Progress, far from consisting in change, depends on retentiveness. Those who cannot remember the past are condemned to repeat it.
—*George Santayana,* The Life of Reason *(1905-06)*

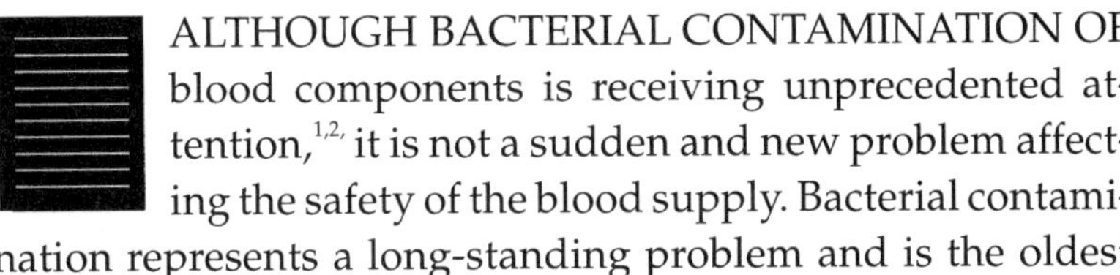

ALTHOUGH BACTERIAL CONTAMINATION OF blood components is receiving unprecedented attention,[1,2] it is not a sudden and new problem affecting the safety of the blood supply. Bacterial contamination represents a long-standing problem and is the oldest transfusion-associated infectious risk.[3] Despite remarkable

---

Roslyn Yomtovian, MD, Director, Blood Bank–Transfusion Medicine, University Hospitals of Cleveland, and Professor, Department of Pathology, Case Western Reserve University School of Medicine, Cleveland, and Elizabeth Palavecino, MD, Fellow, Citywide Blood Bank Fellowship Program, Cleveland, Ohio

advances in reducing the transmission of transfusion-associated infectious agents (primarily viral), bacterial contamination of blood components continues and is proving to be the most difficult transfusion-transmitted disease to eradicate.

While all blood components are susceptible to bacterial contamination, bacterial contamination and transfusion-associated septic reactions are more commonly associated with platelets than with other blood components.[4-6] The main reason for this is that platelet units, stored at room temperature, allow for the growth of most bacteria species; in contrast, Red Blood Cell (RBC) units, stored at 4 C, are able to support growth of only a few bacteria species, most notably, *Yersinia*.[7,8] Indeed, platelet transfusion-associated sepsis is now recognized as the most frequent infectious complication of transfusion therapy—surpassing by up to two orders of magnitude the incidence of transfusion-associated virus transmission.[1,9]

Bacterial contamination of blood presents several challenges that explain, at least in part, why this problem has gone unsolved for over 60 years: 1) First, there has been, as discussed below, lack of widespread recognition of the frequent occurrence of this problem. There is also an incomplete understanding of what constitutes clinically significant contamination and, therefore, what methods need to be developed and implemented to address this problem. This has been especially true in recent years, as viral transfusion-transmissible agents have diverted medical and public attention away from the problem of bacterial contamination. 2) The at-risk patient populations (those receiving the majority of platelet transfusions) frequently exhibit confounding clinical problems that obscure or mask the clinical recognition of transfusion-associated sepsis. In addition, clinical signs and symptoms are highly variable. For example, patients developing bacteremia following transfusion of bacterially contaminated platelets may be asymptomatic, or clinical manifestations may be delayed over an extended period. 3) Bacteria are not generally detectable at the time of donation because they are present in very small numbers, and they continue to grow throughout blood component storage, especially at room temperature. This means that any detection method must be applied and/or interpreted as close to product release as possible rather than at the time of donation. This is a major paradigm shift and presents numerous logistic difficulties reviewed elsewhere in this book. 4) Standard test methods used for virus detection, such as antibody and antigen immunoassays and genetic amplification, are not generally applicable to bacteria detection. Most people have antibodies to bacteria or even fragments of bacteria, reflecting the ubiquitous nature of bacteria. In addition, amplification methods are likely to be contaminated with environmental organisms that are the ones most commonly contaminating blood components. In addition, these methods will detect very small numbers of dead organisms, likely of no clinical concern. 5) Bacteria are remarkably heterogeneous in terms of growth characteristics, optimal means for identification, and clinical implications. Thus, a "standard" or single approach to bacteria detection likely does not apply.

These challenges to confronting and interdicting the problem of bacterial contamination of blood can be more clearly defined and understood (and, hence, can become more readily manageable) through an appreciation of the history and an understanding of the epidemiology of this problem.

History of Bacterial Contamination

Whole Blood, Plasma, and Red Cells

Although, today, platelets are the most common blood component implicated in transfusion-associated sepsis, bacterial contamination predated the modern concept of blood components and was originally recognized as a problem with whole blood, plasma, and serum. Transfusion-transmitted syphilis, first described in 1915,[10] was the first recognized bacterial agent transmitted by blood. It occurred mainly in the setting of direct transfusion between the donor and the recipient via vascular anastomosis, a technique practiced in the early years of the 20th century.[11] Transfusion-transmitted syphilis was virtually eliminated with 1) the ex-vivo (especially refrigerated) storage of blood, 2) the availability of diagnostic testing and specific antibiotic therapy, reducing the frequency of infection, and 3) the application of a donor screening assay beginning in the 1940s.[12] The first edition of the AABB *Standards* published in 1958 required that: "An acceptable serological test for syphilis shall be made on a specimen of the blood. The blood shall not be used for transfusion unless the test is negative. The test is not required if the blood is stored for at least 96 hours prior to use."[13]

Problem of Contamination Recognized with Increased Value of Blood as a Therapeutic Agent

An appreciation, in the contemporary sense, of the potential problem of bacterial contamination of transfused blood dates to 1939 with a seminal publication by Novak in the *Journal of the American Medical Association*. Novak advised that careful attention should be given to the potential for bacterial contamination of stored blood as its use becomes increasingly valuable as a therapeutic agent, admonishing his readers to take this problem more seriously.[14] He pointed out the susceptibility of blood to harbor bacterial contamination, noting an estimated 5% of blood that had been stored for 10 days (in glass bottles), even at 4 to 6 C, was found, on careful examination, to be grossly contaminated. He suggested that the most likely source of contamination is bacteria introduced when the blood is drawn from the donor, noting "Complete sterilization of the skin previous to phlebotomy is impossible, since there are always a few bacteria which escape the bactericidal action of any cutaneous antiseptic. The needle in its course through the skin may encounter these viable organisms, and the chance for introducing them into the bottle with the blood is high." He further noted, with uncanny visionary accuracy, that especially early in storage, "The detection of contamination in stored blood is an uncertain procedure, since the number of organisms is usually small." Novak suggested that the antibiotic sulfanilamide should be added to stored blood to counter, at least temporarily, the in-vitro bacterial growth and, thereby, improve transfusion safety.[14]

The earliest report of a transfusion reaction associated with bacterial contamination of a blood component was made in 1941 by Strumia and McGraw, who described four patients manifesting a severe febrile reaction after transfusion from a pooled lot of liquid plasma, subsequently shown to be contaminated with a large quantity of gram-positive bacilli.[15] All four patients recovered. The authors, acknowledging the risk of bacterial contamination of stored liquid plasma, advocated the use of frozen and/or lyophilized, reconstituted plasma. The first instance of a transfusion reaction associated with bacterial contamination of a unit of whole blood was reported the following year; the recipient died and multiple organisms were isolated from the implicated blood unit.[16]

Differentiation of Epidemiology and Correlation of Organisms with Pathophysiologic Effects

A 1945 report from the Biologics Control Laboratory of the US Public Health Service indicated that bacterial contamination of blood components was clearly a cause for concern.[17] Using a rabbit model, the agency workers studied the pyrogenicity of 28 samples of microorganisms isolated from contaminated blood or plasma. They noted that both gram-negative and gram-positive isolates are able to produce fever when inoculated into rabbits. They noted that gram-negative organisms elicited a slight temperature increase with inocula as low as 2×10^3 to 5×10^3 organisms. A one log greater number of inoculated organisms resulted in a much more marked increase in temperature. Gram-positive organisms, notably the gram-positive cocci, were the least thermogenic of the bacterial inocula and often resulted in a 2- to 3-hour delay in the temperature increase. In some cases, the peak temperature was still not reached for over 6 hours following inoculation. This was the first work to demonstrate a differentiation in the epidemiology of bacterial contamination in blood components on the basis of the type of contaminating organism—gram-positive vs gram-negative, bacilli vs cocci—as well as a correlation between the number of contaminating organisms and the pathophysiologic effects.

In 1951, an article by Borden and Hall published in the *New England Journal of Medicine* described two fatalities associated with gram-negative organisms that were linked to the transfusion of bacterially contaminated preserved whole blood—once again highlighting the clinical importance of this problem.[18] Although it is noted that bacterial growth in stored blood is best controlled by continuous and immediate refrigeration, the authors also noted that in some instances bacterial contamination even in refrigerated stored blood may occur and that "detection of bacterial contamination in stored blood or its products is a problem for which no satisfactory solution has been found." They attributed the probable source of contamination in these specific instances to be unsterile glassware used in the production of blood.

Studies on the Frequency and Clinical Significance of Bacterial Contamination

In the following year, Braude and coworkers studied the frequency and potential clinical significance of bacterial contamination of whole blood.[19] They cultured 1697 consecutive bottles of blood after storage at 4 C for 24 hours and found 2.2% to be contaminated. They noted that bacterial contamination is limited by refrigeration as well as the naturally occurring opsonic properties of blood. The latter was first appreciated and studied by Kolmer[20] in 1939 (who parenthetically suggested the therapeutic efficacy of transfusing fresh blood in patients with septicemia). Braude and coworkers[19] identified coagulase-negative staphylococci as the most common contaminant (19/38 cases), with the authors reiterating that "The entrance of bacteria into some bottles of stored blood appears to be inevitable." The authors, however, struggled with the concept of defining clinically significant contamination. In 36 instances, the contaminated units (identified only retrospectively as culture-positive) were issued for transfusion with only one of them—massively contaminated with diphtheroids—possibly resulting in a delayed septic transfusion reaction. Nonetheless, the concept that skin flora are likely ubiquitous contaminants of donor blood was strengthened by the observation of Gibson and Norris[21] that phlebotomy needles are variably associated with the occurrence of a skin plug that carries a small quantity of bacteria into the donor blood. This solidified the presumption that phlebotomy-associated organisms are the likely source of most instances of bacterial contamination of donor blood.

A further report from the Laboratory of Biologics Control by Pittman[22] in 1953 summarized 18 instances of severe or fatal reactions involving blood or blood components coming to the agency's attention, noting that "This number could be considered as a fraction of the total number that are occurring, since they were heard about incidentally." These 18 instances, spanning the years 1944 through 1952, consisted of one reaction after receipt of serum, 15 reactions after receipt of whole blood, and two reactions after receipt of red cells. All were noted to be gram-negative organisms. In addition to these 18 clinical cases, 29 additional isolates of gram-negative rods and 44 isolates of gram-positive cocci were identified on submitted surveillance cultures. Pittman noted that, overall, it appeared from the data that contamination with gram-positive organisms is more frequent than contamination with gram-negative organisms and that reactions to gram-positive organisms, corroborating the laboratory's earlier work, are generally milder but may be clinically significant at times.

Growth Patterns

In an effort to better understand the clinically evident incidence and magnitude of bacterial contamination of blood components, Geller and Jawetz were the first to demonstrate four growth patterns for bacteria.[23] Each pattern, observed after intentional inoculation of blood with bacteria, demonstrated an initial decrement in the number of bacteria, attributed to naturally occurring opsonic properties. However, following this initial pattern of bacterial reduction, four distinct patterns emerged—immediate log phase growth; somewhat delayed log phase growth; a long plateau (lag) phase following by log phase growth; and a short plateau (lag) phase followed by log phase growth. They noted that the lower the initial contaminating organism content, the greater the likelihood for a prolonged plateau (lag) phase. An understanding of the kinetics of bacterial growth, first demonstrated in this work, has proven essential to current efforts to develop effective strategies to reduce or eliminate the presence of bacteria in stored blood components.

With the emergence of platelet transfusion therapy, the interest in (and the epidemiology of) blood component contamination shifted generally from whole blood, red cells, and plasma to primarily platelets. There was some resurgence of interest in whole blood/red cell bacterial contamination years later with the reports of *Yersinia enterocolitica* contamination first reported in 1982. The epidemiology of this problem (see below) has been monitored carefully by the Centers for Disease Control and Prevention (CDC).[24-26]

Platelets

A 1954 publication ushered in a new era in transfusion therapy. Gardner and coauthors described a procedure for the use of plastic equipment for platelet transfusion and, in particular, noted that the plastic bag and attachments may be prepared and kept sterile indefinitely.[27] This led over the next two decades to approaches for optimizing the use of platelets as a separate blood component. It also eliminated the potential role of improper/incomplete sterilization of glass bottles as a factor in bacterial contamination of stored donor blood. The switch from glass bottles to plastic bags was thus likely instrumental in the changing epidemiology of bacterial contamination of stored donor blood from whole blood, red cells, and plasma to platelets.[28]

The earliest use of platelets involved transfusion immediately or as soon as possible after donor collection. Refrigerated storage was also used, but it was soon realized that platelet function deteriorates rapidly when maintained at 4 C. Work of Murphy and Gardner[27,29] further revolutionized the practice of platelet transfusion therapy by demonstrating maintenance of platelet function during several days of storage at room temperature. They indicated that a "shelf" life of 96 hours would introduce into the use of platelet transfusions a degree of flexibility not possible with refrigerated platelet storage. Although they wisely noted their concern regarding the potential risk of bacterial contamination, they did not believe this to be a problem, on the basis of sampling a small number of units.

Contamination Correlated with Duration of Storage

The potential for a serious problem with bacterial contamination of platelets was emphasized in 1971 with the work of Buchholz and coworkers published in the *New England Journal of Medicine*.[30] This group, noting that the use of platelets stored at room temperature greatly facilitated platelet transfusion therapy, reported two instances of platelet transfusion-transmitted *Enterobacter cloacae* sepsis in two patients after platelet transfusion in July and August 1970. In a pilot study designed to assess the frequency of platelet bacterial contamination, they cultured a 5-mL sample from each of 258 platelet pools comprising a total of 2188 units and demonstrated a unit contamination rate of 2.5%. They cautioned that the high-risk patient populations receiving platelet transfusions are at particular risk for transfusion-transmitted bacterial sepsis. Thus, they warned that room temperature platelet components should be used with caution.

A follow-up investigation by this group designed to further quantitate the extent of platelet bacterial contamination revealed that, in 45 instances (1.4%), 3251 units not subject to pooling were found to contain bacteria on at least one of two plate cultures.[31] In six instances (0.18%), this was confirmed by culture of the identical organism in liquid broth. Most interesting, however, was the observation that the percent of units identified as contaminated was directly correlated with longevity of platelet storage. This suggested for the first time that bacteria entering the donor unit in often undetectable numbers at the time of phlebotomy proliferate throughout the storage period. At about this same time, Goddard and coworkers worried about the potential for proliferation of bacteria in platelet units stored at room temperature.[32] They suggested a then-novel approach to ascertain the potential for contamination by prospective incubation of a sample at 37 C, followed by a Gram's stain on this incubated sample. Unfortunately, follow-up data on the application of this approach are not made available by the authors.

Despite the recognition, in the early 1970s, that platelet bacterial contamination was a variable but recurring problem with room temperature platelets and appeared to correlate with the storage age of the platelets, the clinical utility and convenience of room temperature storage provided momentum to manufacturers for the development of new plastic materials to maintain protracted storage at room temperature. Thus, in 1982 licensure of plastic bags for room temperature platelet storage was extended from 3 to 5 days; in 1984, it was further extended to 7 days. As noted by Dr. Fratantoni, in comments at the February 13, 1986 meeting of the Food and Drug Administration (FDA) Blood Products Advisory Committee (BPAC), this extension of the storage period to 7 days "was based strictly on the functional quality of the platelets and the sterility issue really was not considered at that time."[33] However, in response to an increasing number of reports of platelet bacterial contamination with a predilection for the oldest stored units,[34-36] the FDA BPAC did vote at this February 1986 meeting to reduce the room temperature storage interval of all platelet units to 5 days. They also noted that further data were needed to assess the extent of the problem.

Activity by Federal Agencies and Accrediting Organizations

Because of continuing reports and concern, the topic of platelet bacterial contamination was once again considered by the BPAC in May 1992.[37] In this same year, the CDC reported on four episodes of bacterial contamination of platelet pools, recommending improved surveillance, especially among platelet transfusion recipients experiencing a transfusion reaction. The CDC further recommended that all platelets involved in transfusion reactions be evaluated for bacterial contamination to more accurately estimate the incidence of bacterial contamination of platelets.[38,39] Over time, the focus of the CDC has been on data collection to ascertain the frequency of blood component bacterial contamination associated with transfusion reactions rather than on interdictive strategies. This focus led to the promulgation of the BaCon study (see below).[5,6]

Meanwhile, the FDA convened three workshops to address the ongoing problem of platelet bacterial contamination—September 27, 1995, September 24, 1999, and August 7, 2002.[40-42] At these workshops, much information was presented from national and international perspectives regarding the extent of the problem of platelet bacterial contamination. In addition, industry consultants and representatives presented information regarding a wide array of proposed strategies to reduce, detect, or potentially eradicate platelet bacterial contamination. The approach taken by the FDA has been to encourage the development, by industry, of possible strategies to deal with this problem. Indeed, in February and October, 2002, respectively, the FDA afforded biological device application 510(k) approvals to BacT/ALERT Culture Bottles (bioMérieux, Inc, Durham, NC) and Pall Bacterial Detection System (BDS, Pall Corporation, East Hills, NY) for quality control and sterility testing of leukocyte-reduced platelets. This issue was discussed again by the BPAC on December 12, 2002.[43]

Although no specific practice addresses all of the issues surrounding bacterial contamination, two organizations that promote voluntary standards and assess facilities for compliance are addressing prevention of bacterial contamination of platelets—especially in light of FDA approval of the two culture devices described above. Bacterial contamination of platelets poses a unique challenge in standards-setting because of the variety and complexity of issues, including the short shelf life of platelet components, uncertainty of the optimal sensitivity of the method used, and the type of platelet component being tested. Perhaps the most daunting challenge is that implementation of methods to test for platelet bacterial contamination be balanced with the need to maintain an adequate supply of platelets to meet clinical needs in a timely manner.

The College of American Pathologists modified its Transfusion Medicine Checklist (TRM.44955) to include the question, "Does the laboratory have a system to detect the presence of bacteria in Platelet components?" This is being introduced as a Phase I recommendation.[44] The AABB has provided information on bacterial contamination to its members.[45] Furthermore, the AABB has included a standard in the 22nd edition of its *Standards for Blood Banks and Transfusion Services*[46] to address the problem of bacterial contamination. This standard, effective March 1, 2004, requires methods to limit and detect bacterial contamination in all platelets issued for transfusion.

Epidemiology

As discussed above, bacterial contamination of blood components has been recognized as a serious and ongoing complication of blood transfusion therapy for well over half a century. Lack of appreciation of the clinical significance, lack of clinical recognition, competing priorities, and lack of suitable methods to limit and/or detect bacterial growth have contributed to the persistence of this problem. Currently, as the risks of transfusion-transmitted viral infections have become extremely low, bacterial contamination of blood components has emerged as the most common infectious risk in transfusion medicine.[1,5,9,47]

The true incidence of bacterial contamination of blood components is unknown. The FDA requires reporting of only fatal transfusion-related complications; therefore, the overall incidence of both fatal and nonfatal reactions due to the transfusion of contaminated blood components is significantly underestimated. As stated above, in many instances, bacterial contamination is not suspected as the cause of adverse reaction to transfusion, especially in patients with severe underlying diseases.

Surveillance Data

From 1976 through 1985, the United States FDA reported that of 256 fatalities associated with transfusion, 10% resulted from bacterial contamination of blood components.[48] From 1986 to 1991, 29 (16%) of 182 transfusion-associated fatalities reported to the FDA were caused by bacterial contamination of blood components.[49] From 1998 through 2000, there were 34 confirmed cases of transfusion-transmitted bacterial infection among suspected cases reported to the CDC by blood collection centers participating in the BaCon study. A case was defined as any transfusion reaction meeting clinical criteria in which the same organism species was cultured from a blood component and from recipient blood. Nine of these cases resulted in death. This study also showed that patients at the greatest risk for death received components containing gram-negative organisms.[5] Slightly different numbers of cases were reported in an accompanying report of the evaluation of the reporting system for the BaCon study, with 38 events meeting criteria during the first 2 years; 13 (34%) of 38 were fatal.[6]

Other countries have also evaluated the transfusion-associated bacterial contamination of blood components. In France from 1997 to 1998, 41 of 158 suspected cases involved transfusions of RBCs and 16 involved platelets. Gram-negative rods accounted for nearly half of the bacteria species involved and for all six deaths.[50] In the United Kingdom from 1996 to 1998, from 366 cases of serious complications of blood transfusion reported, 12 were associated with bacterial contamination and one of these was fatal.[51]

Sources of Contamination

Bacterial contamination of blood components can occur during phlebotomy, secondary to the presence of bacteria in the blood of the donor at time of donation, or through contamination of the blood-collecting equipment. Bacteria may also gain entrance into the unit during processing or handling the blood unit following collection.[34,52,53]

In an attempt to reduce the risk of transfusing contaminated blood components, several measures have been recommended. These include exhaustive donor screening to evaluate possible causes for bacteremia, improved disinfection of the skin, diversion or removal of the first 20 to 30 mL of blood collected, optimizing storage temperature, modifications of blood processing including leukocyte reduction, disinfection of the waterbath for thawing frozen products, and more recently, pretransfusion bacteria detection testing.

Bacterial Contamination of Red Cells

As noted above, sepsis associated with the transfusion of bacterially contaminated red cells has been reported very infrequently. However, most reported instances are associated with a high mortality.[3,54] The FDA reported that from 1976 (when mandatory reporting of fatalities began) to 1998, there were 26 deaths related to transfusion of contaminated whole blood or red cells, with an overall risk of less than one fatality per every million units transfused.[3] The most commonly implicated organisms in bacterial contamination of red cells are *Y. enterocolitica*, usually serotype 0:3[55-58] or serotype 0:5,[24] followed by some species of *Serratia* (*S. liquefaciens* or *S. marcescens*) and *Pseudomonas* species. These are all gram-negative organisms, which have the potential of causing endotoxic shock in the recipient. Indeed, patients transfused with RBC units contaminated with these organisms frequently develop high fever and chills during or immediately following transfusion. In addition, these organisms are cryophilic (that is, capable of growth at refrigerator temperatures), and, therefore, they can be present in large numbers, especially in units stored more than 3 weeks, when exponential growth is reached.[7] However, contamination of RBC units with *Y. enterocolitica* has been reported in units stored for only 14 and 16 days.[58,59]

Blood components become contaminated with *Yersinia* species as a result of occult bacteremia in the donor. Contamination of RBC units with *Serratia* or *Pseudomonas* species have been linked mainly to contamination of blood-collecting equipment and waterbaths rather than to donor bacteremia.[60] Nonfermentative gram-negative organisms have also been detected by skin swabs on the arms of up to 11.7% of donors.[61] In addition, it has been demonstrated that there is a significant difference in blood culture contamination rates when skin swabs are procured by personnel specifically trained as phlebotomists compared with personnel not specifically trained as phlebotomists.[62,63]

Contamination with Yersinia enterocolitica

Since the mid-1970s, septicemia caused by transfusion of contaminated RBCs has been reported worldwide. In the United States, the CDC has reported a total of 21 cases of sepsis, in three separate reports, associated with transfusion of RBC units contaminated with *Y. enterocolitica* from November of 1985 to November of 1996.[24-26] *Y. enterocolitica*, a common cause of human infection, is increasing in occurrence and/or recognition. This pathogen can be acquired by ingestion of contaminated food, especially pork or contaminated water. The presence of *Y. enterocolitica* in the blood of donors is always pathogenic; however, overt clinical symptoms are not always present. Symptoms are often mild and include short-duration diarrhea, making it difficult for the donor to remember the episode, especially if happened a week or more before donation.[56,64] Transient *Yersinia* enteritis may be associated with a longer-than-expected period of symptomatic or even asymptomatic bacteremia that causes contamination of donor blood.[65] Fatal *Y. enterocolitica* sepsis associated with red cell contamination has been reported from apparently healthy asymptomatic blood donors.[66] *Y. enterocolitica* contamination has also been reported in autologous donation.[67-69] In fact, autologous blood may be particularly vulnerable to bacterial contamination due to the following: 1) the acceptance of autologous donors is more flexible than that of allogeneic donors, 2) the screening of autologous donors is probably less precise and vigorous compared with the screening of allogeneic donors, and 3) the storage interval for autologous RBC units is typically longer than that for allogeneic units, which maximizes the opportunity for bacterial proliferation.[70]

Recently, a 13-year-old girl developed septic shock after receipt of an autologous RBC transfusion contaminated with *Y. enterocolitica*. Ultimately, she required a bilateral below-the-knee-amputation and developed a seizure disorder—complications attributed to *Y. enterocolitica* sepsis. A few days before the donation, she had complained of abdominal pain and was experiencing mild diarrhea. The authors of this report suggest that for any patient developing shock following any type of transfusion, treatment with aggressive antibiotic therapy should be given until the diagnosis and etiology are known.[71] Transfusion-mediated *Y. enterocolitica* septicemia also has been reported in an adult patient with β-thalassemia.[57] This may correlate, as noted by the authors, with the observation that the growth rate of *Y. enterocolitica*, serotype 0:3 in particular, is in proportion to the amount of iron in the environment.[3] This suggests a potentially important epidemiologic observation given the high incidence of chronically transfused thalassemic patients in Mediterranean countries. It also may have implications for other patients with chronic transfusion requirements. In New Zealand, for reasons not clearly established, the incidence rate of transfusion-transmitted *Yersinia* infection is higher than in other countries and the fatality rate is about 80 times greater than that reported in the United States (one in 104,000 units transfused). This has led one group of investigators to develop a serologic screening test for *Y. enterocolitica.*[72] Investigators have reported that the high incidence rate seen in this area seems to correlate with an increase of *Yersinia* infection seen in this population.[73]

Contamination Involving Other Organisms

Although *Y. enterocolitica* accounts for an estimated 56% of bacterially contaminated RBC units,[74] other organisms have been implicated. *Y. pseudotuberculosis* has the potential of being implicated in contamination of RBC units because the organism can multiply at 4 C.[8] This pathogen is primarily an animal pathogen (domestic and wild animals) and infects humans only occasionally, causing diarrhea and "pseudo appendicitis." Members of the genera *Serratia* are widespread throughout the environment and they are important nosocomial pathogens. *S. marcescens* has been linked to red cell contamination and sepsis following allogeneic as well as autologous blood transfusion.[75,76] In Denmark, *S. marcescens* was implicated in nosocomial septicemia related to contaminated blood transfusion bags. Isolates from three patients, the three units of blood transfused, and the strains isolated at the manufacturer's site were found to be genetically related. The report stated that the incident was interpreted as sporadic and that the contamination occurred during the manufacturing or packaging.[75] Sepsis with a combination of *S. marcescens* and *Pseudomonas aeruginosa* was observed in a patient after receiving two units of autologous blood. One of the units showed abundant growth of both organisms within 24 hours and slight growth of *Staphylococcus epidermidis* within 48 hours of incubation. The source of bacterial contamination could not be identified.[76]

S. liquefaciens, an unusual clinical pathogen, has been increasingly recognized as the cause of transfusion-related sepsis and is associated with a high mortality rate.[60] In a case report, *S. liquefaciens* was isolated from blood bottles probably contaminated during production.[77] The CDC reported five episodes of transfusion-related sepsis and endotoxic shock due to *S. liquefaciens* from July 1992 to January 1999 (four associated with RBC and one with platelet transfusions). Four of the five cases were fatal.[60]

The members of the genera *Pseudomonas* are environmental organisms and can be found in water and soil. They have also been implicated in contamination of blood components. *P. aeruginosa* is the most commonly reported isolate in clinical infections. *P. aeruginosa* has been found as a contaminant of aqueous solutions, such as disinfectant solutions, liquids circulating in dialysis equipment, contact lens solutions, and red cell components.[3] Other Pseudomonas, such as *P. fluorescens* and *P. putida*, are of low virulence and they rarely cause clinical infection; however, they can cause iatrogenic infections associated with the administration of contaminated solutions given their ability to grow at 4 C. *P. fluorescens* has been isolated from skin of 0.3% of blood donors.[61] The cryophilic properties and the potential for transient colonization of skin are two important factors in their ability to cause contamination of RBC units.

Bacterial Contamination of Platelets

As emphasized above, bacterial contamination of blood components, especially platelets, is an important cause of transfusion-associated morbidity and mortality.[5,47,53,78,79] The reported prevalence of bacterial contamination of platelets is highly variable and very difficult to compare. This is because different studies use variable methods of bacteria detection and apply differing case definitions. An estimated 1 in 1000 to 1 in 3000 platelet units (apheresis and whole-blood-derived units) are contaminated with bacteria.[2,79] Transfusion of a contaminated platelet unit is not necessarily associated with a septic transfusion reaction; however, on the basis of reported prevalence rates, it is estimated that a severe episode of transfusion-associated bacterial sepsis occurs in connection with about one-sixth of contaminated platelet units transfused.[79,80] Of 52 cases of bacterial contamination of platelets reported in the literature between 1971 and 1991, 10 were associated with death.[3] Over a 3-year period, 1998 through 2000, from suspected cases reported to the CDC during the BaCon study, the rate of transfusion-transmitted bacteremia (in events/million) was 9.98 for apheresis platelets and 10.64 for whole-blood-derived platelets. The rates of fatal reactions were 1.94 and 2.22, respectively.[5] Overall, the BaCon study estimated a fatality rate of 1 in 500,000 units for apheresis and whole-blood-derived platelets.

In France over a 2-year period, of 16 cases of bacterial contamination associated with platelet transfusion, nine (56%) resulted in severe sepsis or shock. Estimates of the incidence of life-threatening reactions were 9.4 per million (1:106,000) units for whole-blood-derived platelet concentrates and 17.7 per million (1:56,500) for apheresis platelet concentrates.[50]

Most commonly, the organisms implicated in bacterial contamination of platelets are organisms that are part of the normal flora that gain access to the unit during the collection process. Organisms of the normal flora are also known as commensal or endogenous organisms because these organisms become established on a host early in life and persist throughout life. The predominant organisms of the skin flora are Staphylococci (*S. aureus*, coagulase-negative staphylococci), aerobic and anaerobic diphtheroid bacilli (*Corynebacterium, Propionibacterium*), Streptococci, and gram-negative bacilli. Fungi and yeast are often present in skin folds. *S. aureus* and coagulase-negative staphylococci such as *S. epidermidis* are gram-positive cocci and they constitute a major component of the normal flora. Both species are well documented as opportunistic human pathogens and capable of causing severe infections. Members of the genera *Corynebacterium* and

Bacillus are gram-positive rods that are widely distributed in the natural environment and they are usually regarded as contaminants when isolated from clinical specimens. However, these organisms may be opportunistic pathogens and can cause infections in humans if they gain entry into the host tissue or blood through trauma or contaminated blood components.

Sepsis and endotoxic shock due to transfusion of platelets contaminated with *S. liquefaciens* has been reported in two cases. These cases were identified during a look-back investigation of contaminated RBCs, because they had not been linked to the platelet transfusion. This finding demonstrates that contamination of platelet units can be overlooked as the cause of septic reactions.[60]

A 10-year prospective surveillance study performed at the University Hospitals of Cleveland (UHC)[42] found that the most frequently isolated bacteria species from the contaminated platelet units was coagulase-negative staphylococci. Other species detected were *S. aureus, P. aeruginosa, B. cereus, S. marcescens,* and streptococci. Transfusion reactions were identified in 40% of recipients of contaminated units and reactions were not related to a specific organism or to a specific number of organisms, suggesting that one of the main factors involved in the development of transfusion reaction is the underlying condition of the recipient.

Studies at the University Hospitals of Cleveland further demonstrates the value of prospective surveillance in identifying cases of bacterial contamination of platelets compared with that of transfusion-reaction-triggered surveillance used in the BaCon study. One study[81] compared the incidence of bacterial contamination of platelets at UHC using prospective surveillance with that of a neighboring institution using transfusion-reaction-triggered surveillance. Both institutions obtained the majority of their platelets from the same providers. Over a comparable period of time, 14 of 4- and 5-day-old, whole-blood-derived platelets at UHC were bacterially contaminated compared with two cases at the other institution.

Given the transfusion volume at the other institution, if prospective surveillance had been used at that facility, one could have expected 79 to 96 cases. Because many of the patients receiving platelet transfusion are immunosuppressed or neutropenic, septic reactions in these patients are not usually attributed to transfusion of contaminated platelets, as discussed above, and these episodes may not be fully investigated. However, prospective surveillance will identify such cases.[81] Thus, the perceived rate of platelet bacterial contamination is dependent on the detection method used[79,82-84] and the surveillance method (see Fig 1-1). Similarly, while the BaCon study has clearly demonstrated that bacterial contamination is a clinically significant problem, it is limited due to the voluntary par-

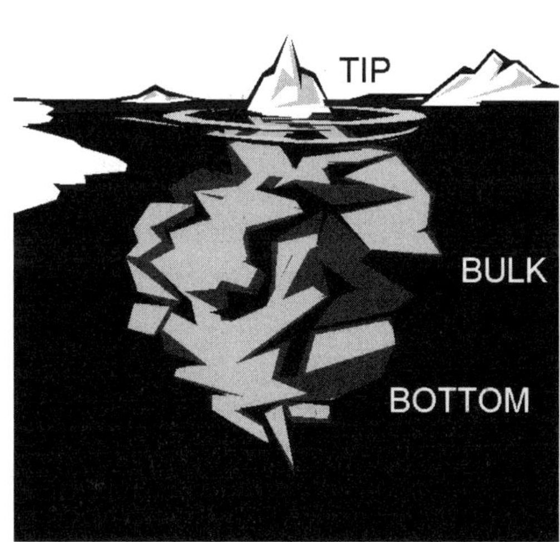

Tip of Iceberg: Contamination identified by transfusion-reaction triggered surveillance – (BaCon Study type analysis)
Bulk of Iceberg: Contamination identified by pretransfusion surveillance – (prospective type analysis)
Bottom of Iceberg: Contamination identified by pretransfusion surveillance or not at all (depends on sensitivity of detection method)

Figure 1-1. Incidence of platelet bacterial contamination depicted as an iceberg.

ticipation and variable expertise in recognizing transfusion-associated sepsis. It is uncertain (but not unanticipated) that many additional cases either did not meet study criteria or were not reported or not recognized. It is possible, indeed likely, as discussed above, that most cases of transfusion of bacterially contaminated units go unrecognized and undetected.

Finally, although it is perhaps assumed that the types of organisms isolated from apheresis units are the same as those isolated from whole-blood-derived units, this may not be the case, over time, as discussed by Dr. Kuehnert at the August 2002 FDA workshop on this topic.[42] Indeed, work from UHC has shown that the epidemiology of platelet bacterial contamination varies, in a statistically significant manner, over time.[85]

With the use of the FDA-approved methods for the detection of bacterially contaminated units, we may have a better understanding of the epidemiology and magnitude of the problem of bacterial contamination of platelets.

Bacterial Contamination of Plasma and Plasma Derivatives

Plasma and plasma derivatives are stored frozen and, therefore, are less likely to be associated with contamination. However, waterbaths used for thawing fresh frozen plasma (FFP) and cryoprecipitate have been reported as contaminated with *Burkolderia cepacia* (formerly *Pseudomonas cepacia)* and *P. aeruginosa*.[86,87] More recently, an outbreak of *P. aeruginosa* in a neonatal intensive care unit, where four newborns were infected or colonized with *P. aeruginosa* within a week, has also been reported. Environmental surveillance and random amplification of polymorphic DNA of the isolates suggested that the outbreak was associated with a contaminated waterbath used to thaw FFP.[88] On the other hand, human serum albumin contains the nutrients needed for bacteria to grow and therefore is a good culture medium. The manufacturing process inactivates viruses but bacteria can still survive. There is a report of endotoxic shock in recipients of specific lots of albumin contaminated with *Pseudomonas* species.[89] The CDC reported

Enterobacter cloacae bloodstream infections traced to contaminated human albumin in two patients from two different states. This multistate outbreak was detected because of prompt reporting and resulted in a worldwide recall of 5%, 20%, 25% albumin, and other plasma derivatives. The epidemiologic and laboratory results seem to suggest that cracks in the glass bottles were responsible for the contamination.[90]

Bacterial Contamination of Stem Cells

Peripheral blood stem cells are being used with increasing frequency to provide hematologic reconstitution. Some centers have evaluated the bacterial contamination of stem cell harvests and found that the incidence of bacterial contamination before cryopreservation ranged from 0.23% to 0.65%[91] in untreated stem cells.[92] This incidence is lower than that reported for marrow harvesting, which has been reported to be 2.1% immediately after collection.[93] After cryopreservation procedures, the bacterial contamination rate may increase by an additional 1%.[94] Investigators have suggested that some of the positive cultures seen after marrow and stem cell collection may be the result of exogenous contamination of blood culture bottles. The organisms usually implicated in contamination of stem cells and marrow products are skin flora, including coagulase-negative staphylococci and alpha hemolytic streptococci. Most studies suggest that despite careful attention to the collection and processing methods, bacteria can be introduced before or during manipulation as well as at thawing. However, no adverse clinical sequelae have been noted following infusion of contaminated products[93-95] because most recipients are receiving antibiotic therapy.

Conclusions

As discussed in this chapter, bacterial contamination of blood components has been and continues to be a serious and ongoing threat to blood transfusion safety. While room-temperature-stored platelets are the most commonly affected component, requiring the most urgent prevention and detection strategies, all blood components are susceptible to bacterial contamination. The growing importance of *Y. enterocolitica* as a human pathogen and its ability to thrive at refrigerated storage temperatures demand, at a minimum, careful ongoing surveillance.

The blood banking and transfusion medicine community is focused on the problem of bacterial contamination. The approval of two systems for bacterial culturing has provided tools to assist in the detection of bacteria in blood components intended for transfusion. The promulgation of voluntary standards that require detection of bacteria underscores the high priority of this problem. With a clearer understanding of transfusion-associated bacterial contamination it is hoped that the newest chapter in the history of this problem will be the final one.

References

1. Goodnough LT, Shander A, Brecher ME. Transfusion medicine: Looking to the future. Lancet 2003;361:161-9.
2. Dodd RY. Bacterial contamination and transfusion safety: Experience in the United States. Transfus Clin Biol 2003;10:6-9.
3. Sazama K. Bacteria in blood for transfusion. A review. Arch Pathol Lab Med 1994;118:350-65.
4. Blajchman MA. Incidence and significance of the bacterial contamination of blood components. Dev Biol 2002;108:59-67.
5. Kuehnert MJ, Roth VR, Haley NR, et al. Transfusion-transmitted bacterial infection in the United States, 1998 through 2000. Transfusion 2001;41:1493-9.
6. Roth VR, Kuehnert MJ, Haley NR, et al. Evaluation of a reporting system for bacterial contamination of blood components in the United States. Transfusion 2001;41:1486-92.
7. Bradley RM, Gander RM, Patel SK, Kaplan HS. Inhibitory effect of 0 degree C storage on the proliferation of *Yersinia enterocolitica* in donated blood. Transfusion 1997;37:691-5.
8. Orozova P, Markova N, Radoucheva T. Properties of *Yersinia enterocolitica* and *Yersinia pseudotuberculosis* in red blood cell concentrate of different ABO groups during 30-day storage at 4 degrees C. Clin Microbiol Infect 2001;7:358-61.
9. Downes KA, Yomtovian R. Advances in pretransfusion infectious disease testing: Ensuring the safety of transfusion therapy. Clin Lab Med 2002;22:475-90.

10. Orton S. Syphilis and blood donors: What we know, what we do not know, and what we need to know. Transfus Med Rev 2001;15:282-91.
11. Schmidt PJ. Syphilis, a disease of direct transfusion. Transfusion 2001; 41:1069-71.
12. Dodd RY. Germs, gels, and genomes: A personal recollection of 30 years in blood safety testing. In: Stramer SL, ed. Blood safety in the new millennium. Bethesda, MD: American Association of Blood Banks, 2001:97-122.
13. Standards for a blood transfusion service. 1st ed. Washington, DC and Chicago: Joint Blood Council, Inc. and American Association of Blood Banks, 1958.
14. Novak M. Preservation of stored blood with sulfanilamide. JAMA 1939;113:2227-9.
15. Strumia MM, McGraw JJ. Frozen and dried plasma for civil and military use. JAMA 1941;116:2378-82.
16. Officer R. Blood storage on active service. Aust N Z J Surg 1942; 12:111-18.
17. Proby TF, Pittman M. The pyrogenicity of bacterial contaminants found in biologic products. J Bact 1945;50:397-411.
18. Borden CW, Hall WH. Fatal transfusion reactions from massive bacterial contamination of blood. N Engl J Med 1951;245:760-5.
19. Braude AI, Sanford JP, Bartlett JE, Mallery OT. Effects and clinical significance of bacterial contaminants in transfused blood. J Lab Clin Med 1952;39:902-16.
20. Kolmer JA. Preserved citrated blood banks in relation to transfusion in the treatment of disease with special reference to the immunologic aspects. Am J Med Sci 1939;197:442.
21. Gibson P, Norris W. Skin fragments removed by injection needles. Lancet 1958;ii:983-5.
22. Pittman M. A study of bacteria implicated in transfusion reactions and of bacteria isolated from blood products. J Lab Clin Med 1953;42:273-88.
23. Geller P, Jawetz E. Experimental studies on bacterial contamination of bank blood. I. The nature of "toxicity" of contaminated blood. J Lab Clin Med 1954;43:696-706.
24. Centers for Disease Control and Prevention. *Yersinia enterocolitica* bacteremia and endotoxin shock associated with red blood cell transfusion—United States, 1987-1988. MMWR Morb Mortal Wkly Rep 1988;37:577-8.
25. Centers for Disease Control and Prevention. Epidemiologic notes and reports update: *Yersinia enterocolitica* bacteremia and endotoxin shock associated with red blood cell transfusions—United States, 1991. MMWR Morb Mortal Wkly Rep 1991;40:176-8.
26. Centers for Disease Control and Prevention. Red blood cell transfusions contaminated with *Yersinia enterocolitica*—United States, 1991-1996, and initiation of a national study to detect bacteria-associated transfusion reactions. MMWR Morb Mortal Wkly Rep 1997;46: 553-5.

27. Gardner FH, Howell D, Hirsch EO. Platelet transfusions utilizing plastic equipment. J Lab Clin Med 1954;43:196-207.
28. Blajchman MA. Transfusion-associated bacterial sepsis: The phoenix rises yet again. Transfusion 1994;34:940-2.
29. Murphy S, Gardner FH. Effect of storage temperature on maintenance of platelet viability—deleterious effect of refrigerated storage. N Engl J Med 1969;280:1094-8.
30. Buchholz DH, Young VM, Friedman NR, et al. Bacterial proliferation in platelet products stored at room temperature. Transfusion-induced Enterobacter sepsis. N Engl J Med 1971;285:429-33.
31. Buchholz DH, Young VM, Friedman NR, et al. Detection and quantitation of bacteria in platelet products stored at ambient temperature. Transfusion 1973;13:268-75.
32. Goddard D, Jacobs SI, Manohitharajah SM. The bacteriological screening of platelet concentrates stored at 22 C. Transfusion 1973;13:103-6.
33. Fratantoni J. Comments at FDA Blood Products Advisory Committee meeting (February 13, 1986). Rockville, MD: CBER Office of Communication, Training, and Manufacturers Assistance, 1986.
34. Braine HG, Kickler TS, Charache P, et al. Bacterial sepsis secondary to platelet transfusion: An adverse effect of extended storage at room temperature. Transfusion 1986;26:391-3.
35. Heal JM, Singal S, Sardisco E, Mayer T. Bacterial proliferation in platelet concentrates. Transfusion 1986;26:388-90.
36. Anderson KC, Gorgone BC, Lew M. Transfusion-related sepsis after prolonged platelet storage (abstract). Blood 1985;66(Suppl):247a.
37. Bacterial contamination. FDA Blood Products Advisory Committee meeting (May 28-29, 1992). Rockville, MD: CBER Office of Communication, Training, and Manufacturers Assistance, 1992.
38. Centers for Disease Control and Prevention. Bacterial contamination of platelet pools—Ohio, 1991. MMWR Morb Mortal Wkly Rep 1992; 41(3):36-7.
39. Zaza S, Tokars JI, Yomtovian R, et al. Bacterial contamination of platelets at a university hospital: Increased identification due to intensified surveillance. Infect Control Hosp Epidemiol 1994;15:82-7.
40. Klein HG, Dodd RY, Ness PM, et al. Current status of microbial contamination of blood components: Summary of a conference. Transfusion 1997;37:95-101.
41. Food and Drug Administration. Workshop on bacterial contamination of platelets (September 24, 1999). Rockville, MD: CBER Office of Communication, Training, and Manufacturers Assistance, 1999. [Available at http://www.fda.gov/cber/minutes/workshop-min.htm.]
42. Food and Drug Administration. Safety and efficacy of methods for reducing pathogens in cellular blood products used in transfusion (August 7-8, 2002). Rockville, MD: CBER Office of Communication, Training and Manufacturers Assistance, 2002. [Available at http://www.fda.gov/cber/minutes/workshop-min.htm.]

43. Bacterial contamination session. FDA Blood Products Advisory Committee meeting, Bethesda, Maryland, December 12, 2002. [Available at http://www.fda.gov/ohrms/dockets/ac/02/briefing/3913b1.htm.]
44. Commission on Laboratory Accreditation. Transfusion medicine checklist (TRM.44955) Phase I. Northfield, IL: College of American Pathologists, 2003. [Available at http://www.cap.org/html/checklist_html/transfusionmedicine_1202.html.]
45. Update on bacterial contamination of platelet units, Association Bulletin #02-8. Bethesda, MD: American Association of Blood Banks, 2002.
46. Fridey JL, ed. Standards for blood banks and transfusion services. 22nd ed. Bethesda, MD: American Association of Blood Banks, 2003:13.
47. Jacobs MR, Palavecino E, Yomtovian R. Don't bug me: The problem of bacterial contamination of blood components—challenges and solutions. Transfusion 2001;41:1331-4.
48. Sazama K. Reports of 355 transfusion-associated deaths: 1976 through 1985. Transfusion 1990;30:583-90.
49. Hoppe PA. Interim measures for detection of bacterially contaminated red cell components. Transfusion 1992;32:199-201.
50. Perez P, Salmi LR, Follea G, et al. Determinants of transfusion-associated bacterial contamination: Results of the French BACTHEM Case-Control Study. Transfusion 2001;41:862-72.
51. Williamson LM, Lowe S, Love EM, et al. Serious hazards of transfusion (SHOT) initiative: Analysis of the first two annual reports. Br Med J 1999;319:16-9.
52. Mertens G, Muylle L, Goossens H. Possible implication of sterile connecting device in contamination of pooled platelet concentrates. Transfus Sci 1997;18:387-92.
53. Blajchman MA. Bacterial contamination and proliferation during the storage of cellular blood products. Vox Sang 1998;74:155-9.
54. Wagner SJ, Friedman LI, Dodd RY. Transfusion-associated bacterial sepsis. Clin Microbiol Rev 1994;7:290-302.
55. Beresford AM. Transfusion reaction due to *Yersinia enterocolitica* and review of other reported cases. Pathology 1995;27:133-5.
56. Haverly RM, Harrison CR, Dougherty TH. *Yersinia enterocolitica* bacteremia associated with red blood cell transfusion. Arch Pathol Lab Med 1996;120:499-500.
57. Roussos A, Stambori M, Aggelis P, et al. Transfusion-mediated *Yersinia enterocolitica* septicemia in an adult patient with beta-thalassemia. Scand J Infect Dis 2001;33:859-60.
58. Jensenius M, Hoel T, Heier HE. [*Yersinia enterocolitica* septicemia after blood transfusion.] Tidsskr Nor Laegeforen 1995;115:940-2.
59. Jones BL, Saw MH, Hanson MF, et al. *Yersinia enterocolitica* septicaemia from transfusion of red cell concentrate stored for 16 days. J Clin Pathol 1993;46:477-8.
60. Roth VR, Arduino MJ, Nobiletti J, et al. Transfusion-related sepsis due to *Serratia liquefaciens* in the United States. Transfusion 2000;40:931-5.

61. Puckett A, Davison G, Entwistle CC, Barbara JA. Post transfusion septicaemia 1980-1989: Importance of donor arm cleansing. J Clin Pathol 1992;45:155-7.
62. Weinbaum FI, Lavie S, Danek M, et al. Doing it right the first time: Quality improvement and the contaminant blood culture. J Clin Microbiol 1997;35:563-5.
63. Schifman RB, Strand CL, Meier FA, Howanitz PJ. Blood culture contamination: A College of American Pathologists Q-Probes study involving 640 institutions and 497134 specimens from adult patients. Arch Pathol Lab Med 1998;122:216-21.
64. McDonald CP, Barbara JA, Hewitt PE, et al. *Yersinia enterocolitica* transmission from a red cell unit 34 days old. Transfus Med 1996;6:61-3.
65. Strobel E, Heesemann J, Mayer G, et al. Bacteriological and serological findings in a further case of transfusion-mediated *Yersinia enterocolitica* sepsis. J Clin Microbiol 2000;38:2788-90.
66. Stubbs JR, Reddy RL, Elg SA, et al. Fatal *Yersinia enterocolitica* (serotype 0:5,27) sepsis after blood transfusion. Vox Sang 1991;61:18-23.
67. Sire JM, Michelet C, Mesnard R, et al. Septic shock due to *Yersinia enterocolitica* after autologous transfusion. Clin Infect Dis 1993;17:954-5.
68. Richards C, Kolins J, Trindade CD. Autologous transfusion-transmitted *Yersinia enterocolitica*. JAMA 1992;268:154-2.
69. Haditsch M, Binder L, Gabriel C, et al. *Yersinia enterocolitica* septicemia in autologous blood transfusion. Transfusion 1994;34:907-9.
70. Yomtovian R. Practical aspects of preoperative autologous transfusion. Am J Clin Pathol 1997;107:S28-35.
71. Benavides S, Nicol K, Koranyi K, Nahata MC. *Yersinia* septic shock following an autologous transfusion in a pediatric patient. Transfus Apheresis Sci 2003;28:19-23.
72. Kendrick CJ, Baker B, Morris AJ, O'Toole PW. Identification of *Yersinia*-infected blood donors by anti-Yop IgA immunoassay. Transfusion 2001;41:1365-72.
73. Theakston EP, Morris AJ, Streat SJ, et al. Transfusion transmitted *Yersinia enterocolitica* infection in New Zealand. Aust N Z J Med 1997;27:62-7.
74. Brecher ME. Bacterial contamination of blood products. In: Simon TL, Dzik WH, Snyder EL, et al, eds. Rossi's principles of transfusion medicine. 3rd ed. Philadelphia: Lippincott Williams & Wilkins, 2002:789- 801.
75. Heltberg O, Skov F, Gerner-Smidt P, et al. Nosocomial epidemic of *Serratia marcescens* septicemia ascribed to contaminated blood transfusion bags. Transfusion 1993;33:221-7.
76. Dinse H, Deusch H. [Sepsis following autologous blood transfusion.] Anaesthesist 1996;45:460-3.
77. Ruden H, Gundermann KO. [Case report of the contamination of preserved blood with *Klebsiella oxytoca* and *Serratia liquefaciens*.] Zentralbl Bakteriol Mikrobiol Hyg [B] 1982;176:444-52.

78. Blajchman MA, Goldman M. Bacterial contamination of platelet concentrates: Incidence, significance, and prevention. Semin Hematol 2001;38:20-6.
79. Yomtovian R, Lazarus HM, Goodnough LT, et al. A prospective microbiologic surveillance program to detect and prevent the transfusion of bacterially contaminated platelets. Transfusion 1993;33:902-9.
80. Blajchman MA. Reducing the risk of bacterial contamination of cellular blood components. Dev Biol Stand 2000;102:183-93.
81. Dykstra A, Hoeltge G, Jacobs MR, et al. Platelet bacterial contamination (PBC) rate is surveillance method dependent (abstract). Transfusion 1999;38(Suppl):104S.
82. Loukhmas L, Houmane N, Mskine M, et al. [Prevalence of bacterial contamination of standard platelet units: Prospective study.] Transfus Clin Biol 2000;7:171-6.
83. AuBuchon JP, Cooper LK, Leach MF, et al. Experience with universal bacterial culturing to detect contamination of apheresis platelet units in a hospital transfusion service. Transfusion 2002;42:855-61.
84. Liu HW, Yuen KY, Cheng TS, et al. Reduction of platelet transfusion-associated sepsis by short-term bacterial culture. Vox Sang 1999;77: 1-5.
85. Dykstra A. Jacobs MR, Yomtovian R. Prospective microbiologic surveillance (PMS) of random-donor (RDP) and single-donor apheresis platelets (SDP)(abstract). Transfusion 1998;38(Suppl):104S.
86. Casewell MW, Slater NG, Cooper JE. Operating theatre water-baths as a cause of pseudomonas septicaemia. J Hosp Infect 1981;2:237-47.
87. Rhame F, McCullough J, Cameron S. *Pseudomonas cepacia* infections caused by thawing of cryoprecipitate in a contaminated water bath (abstract). Transfusion 1979;19:653.
88. Muyldermans G, de Smet F, Pierard D, et al. Neonatal infections with *Pseudomonas aeruginosa* associated with a water-bath used to thaw fresh frozen plasma. J Hosp Infect 1998;39:309-14.
89. Steere AC, Tenney JH, Mackel DC, et al. *Pseudomonas* species bacteremia caused by contaminated normal human serum albumin. J Infect Dis 1977;135:729-35.
90. Wang SA, Tokars JI, Bianchine PJ, et al. *Enterobacter cloacae* bloodstream infections traced to contaminated human albumin. Clin Infect Dis 2000;30:35-40.
91. Webb IJ, Coral FS, Andersen JW, et al. Sources and sequelae of bacterial contamination of hematopoietic stem cell components: Implications for the safety of hematotherapy and graft engineering. Transfusion 1996;36:782-8.
92. Attarian H, Bensinger WI, Buckner CD, et al. Microbial contamination of peripheral blood stem cell collections. Bone Marrow Transplant 1996;17:699-702.
93. Prince HM, Page SR, Keating A, et al. Microbial contamination of harvested bone marrow and peripheral blood. Bone Marrow Transplant 1995;15:87-91.

94. Schwella N, Zimmermann R, Heuft HG, et al. Microbiologic contamination of peripheral blood stem cell autografts. Vox Sang 1994;67:32-5.
95. Schwella N, Rick O, Heuft HG, et al. Bacterial contamination of autologous bone marrow: Reinfusion of culture-positive grafts does not result in clinical sequelae during the posttransplantation course. Vox Sang 1998;74:88-94.

In: Brecher ME, ed.
Bacterial and Parasitic Contamination of Blood Components
Bethesda, MD: AABB Press, 2003

2

Skin Antisepsis and Initial Aliquot Diversion

MINDY GOLDMAN, MD, FRCP(C); JONG-HOON LEE, MD; AND MORRIS A. BLAJCHMAN, MD, FRCP(C)

INADEQUATE DONOR SKIN ANTISEPTIC PREParation has long been recognized as an important contributor to blood component contamination.[1,2] Coagulase-negative *Staphylococci*, *Staphylococcus aureus*, *Corynebacterium*, *Propionibacterium acnes*, and *Bacillus* species that constitute the normal skin flora account for

Mindy Goldman, MD, FRCP(C), Executive Director, Medical Affairs, Donors and Transplantation, Canadian Blood Services, Ottawa, Ontario, Canada; Jong-Hoon Lee, MD, Medical Officer, Office of Blood Research and Review, Center for Biologics Evaluation and Research, Food and Drug Administration, Rockville, Maryland; Morris A. Blajchman, MD, FRCP(C), Professor, Departments of Pathology and Medicine, McMaster University, Head, Transfusion Medicine, Hamilton Regional Laboratory Medicine Program, and Medical Director, Canadian Blood Services, Hamilton, Ontario, Canada

(The views of the authors represent scientific opinions and should not be construed as opinion or policy of the United States Food and Drug Administration or the other

over 90% of all isolates in culture studies of aliquots of whole blood or platelet concentrates.[1,3-5] Although many of these organisms are less pathogenic than endotoxin-producing gram-negative species, skin flora account for a substantial proportion of severe transfusion reactions and fatalities reported to hemovigilance systems. Table 2-1 summarizes the frequency with which various bacteria have been isolated in the UK serious hazards of transfusion (SHOT) hemovigilance program, the French BACTHEM study, and the US Bacterial Contamination (BaCon) study.[6-8] Gram-positive organisms, which are part of normal skin flora, were responsible for 65% of nonfatal reactions and 23% of deaths associated with platelet transfusions as well as 50% of nonfatal reactions and 12% of deaths associated with red cell transfusions.

Platelet transfusions were implicated in 52 fatalities reported to the US Food and Drug Administration (FDA) from 1976 to 1998, of which *S. aureus* and *Staphylococcus epidermidis* accounted for 14 (27%) of the septic deaths (unpublished data). If *Streptococcus* and *Bacillus* species are included among the skin flora, bacteria that make up normal skin flora have been implicated in approximately 40% of the platelet transfusion fatalities reported to the FDA during this period (Table 2-2). However, donor skin may harbor bacteria that are not ordinarily thought of as resident skin flora, including *Clostridia*, *Pseudomonas*, and antibiotic-resistant species.[9-11] The continued, frequent identification of bacterial skin flora associated with transfusion-induced septic episodes compel us to reexamine the possible effectiveness of various donor skin antisepsis methods currently in use at blood centers and the possibility of reduced blood contamination by diversion of the first few mL of donor blood.

Normal Skin Flora

It may not be possible to sterilize the skin without damaging it or without incurring unacceptable adverse systemic effects. The inability to sterilize the skin safely through conventional

Table 2-1. Pathogens Associated with Transfusion-Transmitted Bacteremia or Death (Data from SHOT, BACTHEM, and BaCon Studies)[6-8]

Platelets	Nonfatal Reactions	Fatalities
Gram-positive, normal skin flora		
Coagulase-negative *Staphylococcus*	17	1
Staphylococcus aureus	5	1
Propionibacterium acnes	3	0
Bacillus species	6	1
Subtotal	31 (65%)	
Other gram-positive organisms		3 (23%)
Streptococcus pneumoniae	1	0
Group B *Streptococcus*	3	1
Group G *Streptococcus*	1	0
Subtotal	5 (10%)	1 (8%)
Gram-negative, Enterobacteriaceae		
Escherichia coli	6	2
Serratia species	0	3
Enterobacter species	3	2
Klebsiella species	1	1
Providencia rettgeri	0	1
Yersinia enterocolitica	1	0
Subtotal	11 (23%)	9 (69%)
Other gram-negative organisms		
Acinetobacter species*	1	0
Subtotal	1 (2%)	0 (0%)
Total for platelets	48	13

(continued)

Table 2-1. Pathogens Associated with Transfusion-Transmitted Bacteremia or Death (Data from SHOT, BACTHEM, and BaCon Studies)[6-8] (continued)

Red Cells	Nonfatal Reactions	Fatalities
Gram-positive, normal skin flora		
Coagulase-negative *Staphylococcus*	8	1
Staphylococcus aureus	2	0
Propionibacterium acnes	1	0
Corynebacterium species	2	0
Subtotal	13 (50%)	1 (12%)
Gram-negative, Enterobacteriaceae		
Escherichia coli	2	0
Serratia species	3	3
Enterobacter species	1	1
Klebsiella species	1	0
Proteus species	1	0
Yersinia enterocolitica	1	1
Subtotal	9 (35%)	5 (63%)
Other gram-negative organisms		
Acinetobacter species*	3	1
Pseudomonas species	1	1
Subtotal	4 (15%)	2 (25%)
Total for red cells	26	8

*May be part of normal skin flora.

means is consistent with the distribution of bacterial flora on and within the skin.[12] For the purposes of this discussion, the skin may be regarded as consisting of three structures: 1) an outer epidermal keratin layer, 2) an inner epidermal layer of

Table 2-2. Transfusion-Associated Septic Fatalities Associated with Platelets, Reported to the FDA from 1976 to 1998

Organisms	Number of Cases		Percent of All Reports	
Staphylococcus aureus	9	17%	27%	41%
Staphylococcus epidermidis	5	10%		
Streptococcus species	4	8%	14%	
Bacillus species	3	6%		
Klebsiella species	9	17%		
Serratia species	8	15%		59%
Salmonella species	4	8%		
Pseudomonas species	3	6%		
Enterobacter species	3	6%		
Escherichia coli	3	6%		
Proteus mirabilis	1	2%		
All organisms	**52**		**100%**	

squamous epithelial cells, and 3) a dermal connective tissue layer below the epidermis, which contains hair follicles with associated sweat and sebaceous glands. In simple terms, the inner epidermal layer consists mostly of stacked, irregular, flat cells that are tightly adherent to each other and well suited to resist bacterial entry. Senescent surface cells give rise to the outer keratin layer and are replaced by dividing basal cells.

Based on this simplified view of skin histology, normal skin flora may be classified into three types: 1) transient flora, adherent to the surface of the keratin layer and derived from the environment, 2) surface-resident flora, which probably live and multiply on the surface of the inner epidermal layer, and 3) deep-resident flora, which probably live and multiply deep within the skin, within hair follicles, and associated sweat and sebaceous glands. One can anticipate that the sterilized skin surface is repopulated readily by resident flora emerging from deeper skin layers, particularly with active secretion of sweat and sebum. Richards[13] has reported that bacterial flora repopulation is approximately one-fourth complete in 24 hours before reaching its basal level in about a week and that repopulation occurs more rapidly with sweating, particularly when gloves are worn. Flora repopulation kinetics after skin antisepsis suggests that the optimal antiseptic method for collecting blood from healthy volunteers may be different from methods designed for preoperative use or catheter placement.

Skin Antisepsis

Evaluation of Skin Disinfection Efficacy

Ideally, the evaluation of different skin disinfection methods should be performed in a randomized, controlled trial, with the outcome measure being the positive culture rate of the blood or blood components collected using each method. Unfortunately, given the relative rarity of positive cultures, to our knowledge, only one such study has been performed.[14] Table 2-3 summarizes the relative strengths and weaknesses of the various evaluation methods used, which should be kept in mind when interpreting the data generated by these studies. Another difficulty in interpreting the various studies is the importance of well-trained, experienced personnel to perform skin disinfection. For example, a significant decrease in the blood culture contamination rate may occur after informing staff of their individual contamination rates or after introducing a specialized phlebotomy team.[26,27] Improved results seen with a new disinfection protocol may be due to enhanced staff training and awareness of the importance of skin antisepsis rather than to the merits of a particular protocol. Given the importance of training in the efficacy of this critical step, it would

Table 2-3. Methods of Evaluation of Skin Disinfection Protocols

Method	Selected References	Strengths	Weaknesses
Culture of blood components	Lee et al[14]	• Direct measure of relevant outcome	• Because outcome is rare, studies are difficult to perform
Swab and/or plating technique on skin after disinfection	Goldman et al[15] McDonald et al[16,17] Pleasant et al[18]	• Subject may act as own control before and after disinfection • Different methods can be compared on the same donor • Quantification of bacteria is possible • The same personnel may perform multiple methods • Different methods may be compared, as technique is easy to perform	• Measures surface bacteria only • Surrogate laboratory measure

(continued)

Table 2-3. Methods of Evaluation of Skin Disinfection Protocols (continued)

Method	Selected References	Strengths	Weaknesses
Culture of washing fluid after disinfection	Folléa et al[19] Lilly et al[20]	• Subject may act as own control • Different methods can be compared on the same donor • Quantitation of bacteria is possible • The same personnel may perform multiple methods • Deeper skin flora may be dislodged	• Difficult to perform • Surrogate laboratory measure

Blood culture studies of contamination rates	Schifman et al[21] Strand et al[22] Little et al[23] Calfee et al[24]	• Large-volume phlebotomy sample • Common hospital diagnostic test, large amount of data available	• Collected by hospital personnel under poorly controlled conditions • Definition of contaminated culture variable • Baseline contamination rate highly variable • Bacteria that grow in blood culture media at 37 C may not grow in blood components
Vascular catheter-related septicemia	Chaiyakunapruk et al[25]	• Common hospital procedure, large amount of data available	• Procedure and time course of indwelling catheter are different from blood donation

be useful for blood collection services to be able to perform quality control on donor arm preparation. Contact plate cultures have been used for this purpose in the United Kingdom and Australia, but there is no set standard on the acceptable number of positive cultures or the significance of scanty growth, when observed.[28,29]

Factors Affecting the Efficacy of Skin Disinfection

The factors that may influence the overall effectiveness of a particular antisepsis method are listed in Table 2-4. Washing with soaps and detergents may physically remove bacteria but may not result in bacterial inactivation. Additionally, detergent residue may interfere with the effectiveness of the antiseptics applied subsequent to washing. Therefore, if soap is used for basic hygiene, it must be completely removed before applying an antiseptic. Alcohols, tincture of iodine, iodophors, and chlorhexidine are all effective antiseptic agents that are used currently in various settings such as hospital hand degerming, preoperative antisepsis, or before performing blood cultures or catheter insertion.

Antiseptic Agents

Alcohol is a time-honored skin antiseptic.[12,30] As a class of skin antiseptics, alcohols, in the presence of water, appear to exert their antimicrobial action by protein denaturation. When appropriately diluted, alcohols show excellent activity against most bacteria (gram-positive and gram-negative) as well as good activity against many fungi, but they are not effective against bacterial spores. If properly used, alcohols provide extremely rapid reduction in skin microbial flora and continue to exert their antimicrobial effect for several hours after application. Among the alcohols frequently used in skin antisepsis (ethyl and propyl alcohols), isopropyl alcohol (IPA) may be most desirable for most situations, including blood collection. As a nonpotable alcohol, IPA is not subject to the regulatory restrictions and taxes commonly imposed on ethanol; therefore,

Table 2-4. Factors Affecting Skin Disinfection[12,16,18,21,26,27,30,31]

- Antiseptic used
  - Alcohol
  - Tincture of iodine
  - Povidone-iodine
  - Chlorhexidine
- Concentration of antiseptic
- Multiple vs single antiseptic agents
- Single vs two-step procedure
- Method of application of antiseptic—scrub, swab, ampule, applicator
- Contact time between the antiseptic and the skin
- Training and expertise of personnel

it is less expensive and more readily available than ethanol. IPA also appears to be more effective than ethanol against bacteria and lipid-enveloped viruses, possibly because of its increased ability to solubilize fats, but at the expense of increased skin drying and roughness, particularly when used frequently.

Tincture of iodine, usually formulated as 1% to 2% iodine and potassium iodine in 70% alcohol, exerts a microbicidal effect by cell wall penetration, oxidation, and substitution of microbial contents with free iodine.[12,30] Iodine has a wide range of activity against both gram-positive and gram-negative bacteria and fungi, as well as some activity against bacteria spores. Iodophors, such as povidone-iodine, are complexes that consist of iodine and a carrier molecule such as polyvinylpyrrolidone. Formulations of 7.5% or 10% povidone-iodine usually contain 0.75% and 1% free iodine, respectively. Although iodophors may cause less skin irritation and fewer allergic reactions than tincture of iodine, they also have a slower onset of antimicrobial action because free iodine must be released from the carrier complex over time.[32] This may be important in the setting of a busy blood donor clinic.

Chlorhexidine gluconate causes disruption of microbial cell membranes and precipitation of cell contents.[12,30] It is usually formulated as a 0.5% to 1% solution in alcohol or as a 0.5% to 2% aqueous solution. It has greater activity against gram-positive bacteria compared with gram-negative bacteria and is ineffective against spores. Chlorhexidine has strong affinity for the skin, and its antibacterial effect persists for many hours after application.[33,34] This may be particularly important for procedures such as catheter placement, but less relevant for blood donation. Chlorhexidine causes little skin irritation and is often used for blood donors who are allergic to iodine.[35]

Multiple vs Single Agents for Skin Preparation

The use of multiple antiseptic agents, either in single or in multiple application steps, has been accepted generally as good clinical practice. This practice has carried over to blood collection from healthy volunteers.[36] Presumably, the use of multiple agents that possess different mechanisms of antimicrobial action results in an overall synergistic effectiveness of a given antisepsis method. The results obtained by Lilly et al and others, however, suggest that the use of multiple agents does not necessarily result in bacterial reduction beyond that achievable through the use of single agents.[20]

Method of Application of Antiseptic

The way in which an antiseptic is applied to the skin is as important as the choice of the agent itself.[16,18,21] In most protocols, an initial "scrub" step is used to provide both the physical removal of desquamated epidermis as well as microbial killing. The second "prep" step usually involves careful application of the disinfectant, starting at the site of venipuncture.[35] In some studies, kits that contain sponge brushes for the scrub step and ampules for the disinfection step were more effective than swabs.[16,18,21] Adequate application time and the drying of the antiseptic before initiating the phlebotomy appear to be important steps to achieve optimal disinfection.[16]

Training and Expertise of Personnel

As previously mentioned, the use of a dedicated phlebotomy team, or enhanced staff training and feedback on performance, can have a marked effect on the contamination rate in blood culture studies.[26,27,31] These issues are equally critical for blood collection personnel.

Comparison of Disinfection Protocols

Studies comparing skin disinfection protocols are summarized in Table 2-5. Only studies published since 1990 that provided sufficient information about the concentration of antiseptic agents and the method of application used were included.[14-16,21-25] In addition, a Q probe study by the College of American Pathologists found that lower blood culture contamination rates were associated with use of a dedicated phlebotomy service and use of tincture of iodine for skin disinfection.[31] A case control study by Perez et al found that repetition of a scrub with a gauze pad before the "prep" phase of disinfection was associated with lower bacterial contamination of whole blood donations.[37] Of note, the scrub phase in this study was only 5 to 10 seconds, as opposed to the 30 seconds required by most manufacturers of disinfection kits, the protocols in the AABB *Technical Manual*, and FDA-approved methods of arm preparation.[35,36] Although not all study results are concordant, the following factors appear to be associated with superior disinfection: use of a two-stage method; use of a kit containing a sponge scrub followed by an ampule, rather than swabs or gauze pads; and use of tincture of iodine and alcohol rather than povidone-iodine. The AABB *Technical Manual* details a two-stage procedure involving a 30-second scrub with a 0.7% aqueous iodophor compound, followed by a 10% iodophor compound, applied in a concentric spiral.[35] The preparation solution should be allowed to dry for 30 seconds after application. Methods containing chlorhexidine gluconate and isopropyl alcohol are recommended for donors who are allergic to iodine. In Canada, a two-stage method in-

Table 2-5. Comparison of Disinfection Protocols

Study Design	Protocols Compared	Conclusions and Comments
Lee et al[14]		
2 consecutive protocols used in routine blood collection, culture of platelet pools (n = 18,000 pools in each group)	• 0.5% cetrimide/0.05% CH aqueous solution scrub, 70% IPA • 10% PI scrub, 70% IPA	• 10% PI scrub, 70% IPA superior • Cetrimide not commonly used, weak CH solution
Goldman et al[15]		
Contact plates, different method each arm of same donor (n = 30 to 126 in each group)	• 70% IPA scrub, 2% TI ampule • 7.5% PI swabstick, 10% PI swabstick • 0.5% CH/70% IPA sponge scrub, 0.5% CH/ 70% IPA ampule • Green soap sponge, IPA swab	• 70% IPA scrub, 2% TI ampule superior • Green soap, IPA swab ineffective, 2 other methods equivalent

McDonald et al[16]		
Direct swab and plating, pre- and post-disinfection counts compared (n = 100 each group)	• 0.5% CH/70% IPA wipe X 1 or X 2 • 0.5% CH/0.125% HP/70% IPA scrub X 1 • 70% IPA sponge scrub, 2% TI ampule • 70% IPA sponge scrub, 70% IPA ampule • 7.5% PI swabstick, 10% PI swabstick • 7.5% PI swabstick, 70% IPA swabstick • 70% IPA swabstick X 2	• Marked differences between methods • 2 stage application methods superior • 70% IPA sponge scrub, 2% TI ampule best method • TI must be applied for 30 seconds for best results • Method of application important: scrub superior to wipe or swabstick
Schifman et al[21]		
Blood cultures, randomized trial (n = 770 per method)	• 70% IPA swab, 10% PI swab • 70% IPA/10% acetone scrub, 10% PI ampule	• 70% IPA/10% acetone scrub, 10% PI ampule superior (2.2% vs 4.6% contamination rate) • Method of application important: scrub and ampule superior to swab

(continued)

Table 2-5. Comparison of Disinfection Protocols (continued)

Study Design	Protocols Compared	Conclusions and Comments
Strand et al[22]		
Blood cultures, methods used in alternating time periods (n = 4230 per method)	• 10% PI pad X 3 • 2% TI/47% ethanol pad X 3	• 2% TI/47% ethanol pad superior (3.74% vs 6.25%) • Higher concentration of available iodine plus combination with ethanol in superior method
Little et al[23]		
Blood cultures, randomized trial (n = 1900 per method)	• 70% IPA scrub, 2% TI/47% ethanol ampule • 70% IPA gauze pad, 10% PI gauze pad	• 70% IPA scrub, 2% TI/47% ethanol superior (2.4% vs 3.8%) • Scrub, higher concentration of available iodine, plus combination with ethanol in superior method

Calfee et al[24]		
Blood cultures randomized trial (n = 3100 per method)	• 10% PI swab X 3 • 2% TI/47% ethanol swab X 3 • 10% PI/70% ethyl alcohol swab X 3 • 70% IPA swab X 3	• No statistically significant differences (range, 2.46% to 2.93%) • Minimum delay of 1 minute after 3rd application before cultures
Chaiyakunapruk et al[25]		
Vascular catheter infections meta-analysis of 8 randomized controlled trials (total n = 4143)	• 10% PI • 0.5% to 2% CH in aqueous or alcoholic solution	• CH superior (1% vs 2%) • Longer duration of antimicrobial effect may be important

CH = chlorhexidine; TI = tincture of iodine; IPA = isopropyl alcohol; PI = povidone-iodine; HP = hydrogen peroxide; X 1 = applied once; X 2 = applied twice; X 3 = applied three times.

volving a 70% isopropyl alcohol scrub followed by a 2% iodine tincture solution has been utilized for several years with good donor acceptance.[15]

Bacterial Contamination of Antiseptic Solutions

Bacteria may contaminate antiseptic solutions themselves. Organisms that are found in water or are ubiquitous in the environment, such as *Pseudomonas aeruginosa* and *Pseudomonas fluorescens*, have been detected in solutions of povidone-iodine, dilute benzalkonium chloride, and chlorhexidine gluconate.[38-41] Recently, commercial skin antiseptic kits containing various disinfectants produced by one US manufacturer were recalled because of contamination with multiple bacteria species.[42] In an unrelated incident, a severe septic transfusion reaction due to *P. fluorescens* was traced back to the use of contaminated moistened cool cloths placed on top of the sterile gauze pad on the phlebotomy site during donation.[43] Manufacturers' recommendations must be followed for the preparation and storage of antiseptic solutions, and collection procedures must be carefully controlled to avoid such episodes.

Initial Aliquot Diversion

In spite of adequate surface disinfection, the deeper layers of skin, the subcutaneous hair follicles, and the sebaceous glands may continue to harbour bacteria. In the case of one frequent blood donor associated with regularly contaminated platelet apheresis units, Anderson et al demonstrated that after skin disinfection, surface skin cultures were negative, while blood cultures were positive for coagulase-negative *Staphylococci.*[44] The blood cultures had been taken from an area of skin dimpling in the antecubital fossa, where multiple needle punctures had resulted in scarring of the skin. In an elegant set of experiments performed by Gibson and Norris in 1958, a core of skin tissue was often detected in the needle after most skin punctures.[45] Unfortunately, these experiments have not been repeated with more modern needle designs.

Olthuis et al hypothesized that bacteria associated with venipuncture would more likely be present in the first few milliliters of donor blood.[46] A 2% contamination rate was detected in the first tube of blood collected through an adapter after venipuncture, whereas no contamination could be demonstrated in the second tube. These experiments were performed using an open system plasmapheresis kit; therefore, they are not exactly analogous to platelet apheresis or whole blood collection systems currently in use.

Experimental Models of Diversion

Experimental models have been developed to simulate the distribution of bacteria in fluid passing through a contaminated needle. Figueroa et al introduced a small inoculum of *S. aureus* into a standard collection needle, which was then used to obtain five sequential 5-mL samples from a plasma unit.[47] Experiments were performed using a wet inoculum, or after the inoculum had dried in the lumen. In either case, the majority of the bacteria were cultured from the first two samples (10 mL) of plasma. There was a 1- to 2-log decrease in the number of bacteria cultured from the fifth 5-mL aliquot compared to that seen in the first 5-mL aliquot of plasma. In a slightly different model system, Wagner et al inserted a collection needle into a whole blood or sterile saline bag through a medication site that had been heavily contaminated with *S. aureus* and allowed to dry.[48] Quantitative bacterial cultures were then performed on six successive 7-mL samples drawn through a diversion arm, followed by a 40-mL sample drawn into a transfer pack. In both the saline and whole blood experiments, bacterial colony counts were highest in the first 7-mL tube and decreased in each subsequent tube. In the whole blood experiments, 88% of the total *S. aureus* load was present in the first three tubes, with 95% present in the six tubes. Diversion of the first 21 to 42 mL of blood therefore resulted in a 1-log decrease in the organism. However, the high level of contamination of the medication site, although allowing accurate quantitation of bacteria, does not reflect the low level of residual contamination expected on donor skin after disinfection.

Contamination Rate of Diverted Samples

Expanding on the initial observations of Olthuis, Bruneau et al used a closed whole blood collection system designed for the diversion of two separate 15-mL samples after venipuncture.[49] Both aerobic and anaerobic cultures were performed on the diverted samples, using the automated BacT/ALERT system (bioMérieux, Durham, NC). The four different French collection regions participating in the study had different skin disinfection protocols and differed widely in their bacterial contamination rates. Overall, bacteria were detected in one or both of the samples in 76 of 3385 donations (2.2%). In 74% of contamination cases, bacteria were present in the first sample only. Coagulase-negative *Staphylococci* and other gram-positive cocci accounted for 81% of bacterial species detected, followed by *P. acnes* and other gram-positive bacilli in 13.9% of cases and gram-negative bacilli in only 5.1% of cases. No platelet concentrates were prepared from these whole blood donations; however, 53 plasma units and 61 red cell units associated with positive culture samples were retrieved. None of the plasma units and 7 of the red cell units (11%) also had positive cultures. Although the numbers are small, contaminated red cell units were more common in cases where both samples were positive, perhaps indicating a higher initial bacterial load. The overall contamination rate of 2.2% found in whole blood samples in this study is very high, compared with contamination rates found in studies of blood components (ie, platelets). It is probable that not all bacteria that are inoculated into the whole blood collection set survive or proliferate to sufficiently high levels during component storage to cause a septic transfusion reaction. Therefore, although promising, these results cannot be extrapolated directly to estimate the efficacy of initial diversion on the reduction of the clinically relevant bacterial contamination associated with the transfusion of blood components.

Bacterial Contamination Rates After the Introduction of Diversion

Three studies, summarized in Table 2-6, have measured bacterial contamination rates before and after the introduction of diversion of 10 to 42 mL of blood. de Korte et al used a sampling bag with integrated needles to perform 10-mL aerobic and anaerobic cultures of whole blood stored on butane-1, 4-diol cooling plates before component production.[4] A highly significant decrease in the rate of positive cultures was noted after initiation of diversion of the first 10 mL of blood. This was particularly striking for coagulase-negative *Staphylococcus*, which decreased from 0.14% to 0.03% of collections after introduction of initial diversion. Similar preliminary results have been reported by McDonald.[52] The studies by Bos et al and Schneider et al indicate a statistically significant decrease in the rate of contamination of buffy coat pooled platelets after introduction of collection sets with initial diversion.[50,51]

In summary, data from both laboratory and clinical studies demonstrate a decrease in bacterial contamination with initial diversion of the first few milliliters of blood. Although initial diversion of 10 mL is beneficial, diversion of over 30 mL may be optimal. Several manufacturers have developed collection sets with a "Y" configuration that permit the initial diversion of up to 42 mL of blood. After filling the diversion pouch, the tubing is clamped to prevent back-flow. An obdurator is then broken on the other limb of the "Y" to permit filling of the main collection bag. Samples needed to perform blood grouping and infectious disease testing are taken from the diversion pouch. The diversion pouch has been mandatory in France since 2000 and is used extensively in The Netherlands, Belgium, the United Kingdom, and other European countries.[53] Although not required by regulatory agencies, collection sets

Table 2-6. Evaluation of the Effect of Initial Aliquot Diversion on the Subsequent Bacterial Contamination Rate of Blood Components

Study	Volume of Diversion	Component Cultured	Time from Phlebotomy to Culture	Positive Cultures/Total Cultures (%)	
				Without Diversion	With Diversion
de Korte et al[4]	10 mL	Whole blood	2-14 hours	63/18,257 (0.35)	15/7,087 (0.21)
Bos et al[50]	20 mL	Buffy coat pools	Not stated*	42/4,064 (1.03)	7/1,447 (0.48)
Schneider et al[51]	42 mL	Buffy coat pools	Over 5 days†	14/602 (2.32)	4/409 (0.98)

*Cultures done during pooling of five buffy coat platelet concentrates.

†Outdated pools of four buffy coat platelet concentrates.

with a diversion pouch have been licensed in both the United States and Canada. Both Canadian blood suppliers have introduced diversion pouch methodology during 2003.

Conclusions

It is important to note that the 22nd edition of the AABB *Standards for Blood Banks and Transfusion Services* includes a standard stating that "The blood bank or transfusion service shall have methods to limit and detect bacterial contamination in all platelet components."[54] Which methods conform to this standard will need to be established. Relevantly, both improved skin disinfection techniques and the use of an initial diversion system are methods that could reduce the risk of the bacterial contamination of blood products. However, the extent of reduction to be achieved by these two interventions is difficult to predict at this time.

The reduction in transfusion-associated septic risk achieved by improving skin disinfection and/or initial aliquot diversion is likely to be modest. This is because the majority (greater than 60%) of reported clinically evident transfusion-associated septic episodes are not due to bacteria species that can be classified as skin flora. Nonetheless, these two interventions (improved skin disinfection and initial aliquot diversion) are interim measures that should be considered until the institution of completely effective bacteria detection and/or pathogen reduction systems.

References

1. Goldman M, Blajchman MA. Bacterial contamination. In: Popovsky M, ed. Transfusion reactions. 2nd ed. Bethesda, MD: AABB Press, 2001:129-54.
2. Puckett A, Davison G, Entwistle CC, Barbara JAJ. Post transfusion septicaemia 1980-1989: Importance of donor arm cleansing. J Clin Pathol 1992;45:155-7.
3. de Korte D, Marcelis JH, Soeterboek AM. Determination of the degree of bacterial contamination of whole-blood collections using an automated microbe-detection system. Transfusion 2001;41:815-18.

4. de Korte D, Marcelis JH, Verhoeven AJ, Soeterboek AM. Diversion of first blood volume results in a reduction of bacterial contamination for whole-blood collections. Vox Sang 2002;83:13-16.
5. Soeterboek AM, Welle FHW, Marcelis JH, et al. Sterility testing of blood products in 1994/1995 by three cooperating blood banks in The Netherlands. Vox Sang 1997;72:61-2.
6. Serious Hazards of Transfusion (SHOT) annual report 2000-2001. [Available at www.shot.demon.co.uk/reports.]
7. Perez P, Salmi LR, Folléa G, et al. Determinants of transfusion-associated bacterial contamination: Results of the French BACTHEM case-control study. Transfusion 2001;41:862-72.
8. Kuehnert MJ, Roth VR, Haley NR, et al. Transfusion-transmitted bacterial infection in the United States, 1998 through 2000. Transfusion 2001;41:1493-9.
9. McDonald CP, Hartley S, Orchard K, et al. Fatal *Clostridium perfringens* sepsis from a pooled platelet transfusion. Transfus Med 1998;8:19-22.
10. Stenhouse MA, Milner LV. A survey of cold-growing gram-negative organisms isolated from the skin of prospective blood donors. Transfus Med 1992;2:235-7.
11. Sapatnekar S, Wood EM, Miller JP, et al. Methicillin-resistant *Staphylococcus aureus* sepsis associated with the transfusion of contaminated platelets: A case report. Transfusion 2001;41:1426-30.
12. Larson EL. APIC guidelines for infection control practice. Am J Infect Control 1995;23:251-69.
13. Richards RC. Some practical aspects of surgical skin preparation. Am J Surg 1963;106:575-85.
14. Lee CK, Ho PL, Chan NK, et al. Impact of donor arm skin disinfection on the bacterial contamination rate of platelet concentrates. Vox Sang 2002;83:204-8.
15. Goldman M, Roy G, Fréchette N, et al. Evaluation of donor skin disinfection methods. Transfusion 1997;37:309-12.
16. McDonald CP, Lowe P, Roy A, et al. Evaluation of donor arm disinfection techniques. Vox Sang 2001;80:135-41.
17. McDonald CP, Roy A, Majahan P, et al. Evaluation of the chloraprep disinfection system (abstract). Vox Sang 2002;83(Suppl 2):5.
18. Pleasant H, Marini J, Stehling L. Evaluation of three skin preps for use prior to phlebotomy (abstract). Transfusion 1994;34(Suppl):14S.
19. Folléa G, Saint-Laurent P, Bigey F, et al. Evaluation bactériologique quantitative d'une méthode de désinfection cutanée chez les donneurs de sang. Transfus Clin Biol 1997;4:523-31.
20. Lilly HA, Lowbury EJL, Wilkins MD. Limits to progressive reduction of resident skin bacteria by disinfection. J Clin Pathol 1979;32:382-5.
21. Schifman RB, Pindur A. The effect of skin disinfection materials on reducing blood culture contamination. Am J Clin Pathol 1993;99:536-8.
22. Strand CL, Wajsbort RR, Sturmann K. Effect of iodophor vs iodine tincture skin preparation on blood culture contamination rate. JAMA 1993;269:1004-6.

23. Little JR, Murray PR, Traynor PS, Spitznagel E. A randomized trial of povidone-iodine compared with iodine tincture for venipuncture site disinfection: Effects on rates of blood culture contamination. Am J Med 1999;107:119-25.
24. Calfee DP, Farr BM. Comparison of four antiseptic preparations for skin in the prevention of contamination of percutaneously drawn blood cultures: A randomized trial. J Clin Microbiol 2002;40:1660-5.
25. Chaiyakunapruk N, Veenstra DL, Lipsky BA, Saint S. Chlorhexidine compared with povidone-iodine solution for vascular catheter–site care: A meta-analysis. Ann Intern Med 2002;136:792-801.
26. Gibb AP, Hill B, Chorel B, Brant R. Reduction in blood contamination rate by feedback to phlebotomists. Arch Pathol Lab Med 1997;121: 503-7.
27. Weinbaum FI, Lavie S, Danek M, et al. Doing it right the first time: Quality improvement and the contaminant blood culture. J Clin Microbiol 1997;35:563-5.
28. Colville V, Hawker J, Cummings B, Wood E. A role for alcohol in blood service procedures: Considerations for topical application (abstract). Transfusion 2002;42(Suppl):41S.
29. Kitchen AD, Howe PHJ. Donor arm swabbing—how clean is clean? (abstract) Transfus Med 1995;5(Suppl):50.
30. McDonnell G, Russel AD. Antiseptics and disinfectants: Activity, action, and resistance. Clin Microbiol Rev 1999;12:147-79.
31. Schifman R, Strand C, Meir F, Howanitz P. Blood culture contamination: A College of American Pathologists Q-probes study involving 640 institutions and 497,134 specimens from adult patients. Arch Pathol Lab Med 1998;122:216-21.
32. Dykes PJ, Marks R. An evaluation of the irritancy potential of povidone iodine solutions: Comparison of subjective and objective assessment techniques. Clin Exp Dermatol 1992;17:246-9.
33. Hibbard JS, Mulberry GK, Brady AR. A clinical study comparing the skin antisepsis and safety of ChloraPrep, 70% isopropyl alcohol, and 2% aqueous chlorhexidine. J Infus Nurs 2002;25:244-9.
34. Hibbard JS. Administration of 2% chlorhexidine gluconate in 70% isopropyl alcohol is effective in 30 seconds. Infect Control Hosp Epidemiol 2002:23:233-4.
35. Brecher ME, ed. Technical manual. 14th ed. Bethesda, MD: American Association of Blood Banks, 2002:734-5.
36. Recall of sterile povidone iodine, tincture of iodine, benzoin tincture, acetone alcohol, and alcohol antiseptic products as well as sterile Cliniguard® protective dressing, and specified lots of nonsterile products. [Available at http://www.fda.gov_Hlt38182272_Hlt38182273mBM_2_BM_3_edwatch/safety/2000/clinip.htm.]
37. Perez P, Bruneau C, Chassaigne M, et al. Multivariate analysis of determinants of bacterial contamination of whole-blood donations. Vox Sang 2002;82:55-60.

38. Berkelman RL, Lewin S, Allen JR, et al. Pseudobacteremia attributed to contamination of povidone-iodine with *Pseudomonas cepacia*. Ann Intern Med 1981;95:32-6.
39. Oie S, Kamiya A. Microbial contamination of antiseptics and disinfectants. Am J Infect Control 1996;24:389-95.
40. Garcia-Erce JA, Grasa JM, Solano VM, et al. Bacterial contamination of blood components due to *Burlcholderia cepacia* contamination from chlorhexidine bottles. Vox Sang 2002;83:70-1.
41. Panlilio AL, Siegel J, Clark NC, et al. Infections and pseudoinfections due to povidone-iodine solution contaminated with *Pseudomonas cepacia*. Clin Infect Dis 1992;14:1078-83.
42. FDA issues urgent follow-up memo on Clinipad skin preparation recall. AABB Weekly Report 2000;6(13):1-2.
43. Chaffin DJ, Kuehnert MJ. *Pseudomonas fluorescens*-related septic transfusion reaction resulting from contaminated cold cloths (abstract). Transfusion 2002;42(Suppl):41S.
44. Anderson KC, Lew MA, Gorgone BC, et al. Transfusion-related sepsis after prolonged platelet storage. Am J Med 1986;81:405-11.
45. Gibson T, Norris W. Skin fragments removed by injection needles. Lancet 1958;ii:983-5.
46. Olthuis H, Puylaert C, Verhagen C, Valk L. Method for removal of contamination bacteria during venipuncture. Presented at the Fifth International Society for Blood Transfusion Regional Congress, Venice, Italy, July 2-5, 1995.
47. Figueroa PI, Yoshimori R, Nelson E, et al. Distribution of bacteria in fluid passing through an inoculated collection needle (abstract). Transfusion 1995;35(Suppl):11S.
48. Wagner SJ, Robinette D, Friedman LI, Miripol J. Diversion of initial blood flow to prevent whole-blood contamination by skin surface bacteria: An *in vitro* model. Transfusion 2000;40:335-8.
49. Bruneau C, Perez P, Chassaigne M, et al. Efficacy of a new collection procedure for preventing bacterial contamination of whole-blood donations. Transfusion 2001;41:74-81.
50. Bos H, Yedema TH, Luten M, et al. Reduction of the incidence on bacterial contamination by pre-donation drawing blood for safety tests. Vox Sang 2002;83(Suppl 2):014.
51. Schneider T, Tunez V, Fontaine O, et al. Benefits of the pre-donation sampling pouch in order to reduce bacterial contamination of pooled platelets concentrates. Vox Sang 2002;83(Suppl 2):162.
52. McDonald CP. Strategies to reduce transfusion transmission of bacterial infections (abstract). Transfus Med 2002;12(Suppl 1):S13.
53. Andreu G, Morel P, Forestier F, et al. Hémovigilance network in France: Organization and analysis of immediate transfusion incident reports from 1994 to 1998. Transfusion 2002;42:1356-64.
54. Fridey JL, ed. Standards for blood banks and transfusion services. 22nd ed. Bethesda, MD: American Association of Blood Banks, 2003:13.

In: Brecher ME, ed.
Bacterial and Parasitic Contamination of Blood Components
Bethesda, MD: AABB Press, 2003

3

Bacteria Detection

MARLA C. BRUMIT, MD; SHAUNA N. HAY, MT(ASCP); AND MARK E. BRECHER, MD

SEVERAL DIVERSE METHODS TO SCREEN BLOOD components for bacterial contamination are under investigation. Most of the systems under investigation emphasize platelets, which are stored at 20 to 24 C (making an excellent bacterial growth medium), as this component is felt to carry the greatest risk of bacterial overgrowth. Several systems for detecting platelet bacterial contamination are already in use within selected areas of the United States

Marla C. Brumit, MD, Fellow, Transfusion Medicine, Transplantation and Transfusion Services, McLendon Clinical Laboratories; Shauna N. Hay, MT(ASCP), Research Technologist, Transplantation and Transfusion Services, McLendon Clinical Laboratories; and Mark E. Brecher, MD, Director, Transplantation and Transfusion Services, McLendon Clinical Laboratories, University of North Carolina Hospitals, and Professor of Pathology and Laboratory Medicine, University of North Carolina at Chapel Hill, Chapel Hill, North Carolina and Europe. In Belgium and The Netherlands, culturing of platelets is mandatory and, although not required, is commonplace in Sweden, Norway, and Denmark. Additionally, within the United Kingdom, Germany, and Canada, select centers are also screening platelets for bacterial contamination.[1] Diverse culture methods, microscopic examination (eg, Gram's stain), and multireagent strips are generally available and routinely used by some institutions for bacterial screening. Other less widely implemented detection methods, many still under investigation, range from visual inspection for platelet swirling to myriad molecular techniques.

In 2002, the US Food and Drug Administration (FDA) approved two culture techniques (BacT/ALERT, bioMérieux, Durham, NC and BDS, Pall Corporation, East Hills, NY) for in-run quality control of platelets.[2] Recently, the College of American Pathologists (CAP) Commission on Laboratory Accreditation has added a question to the Transfusion Medicine Checklist to assess the presence of a laboratory system to detect bacteria in platelet components. Noncompliance with this standard is classified as a Phase I or minor deficiency.[3] Similarly, the American Association of Blood Banks (AABB) has announced a new standard for blood banks and transfusion services that states "the blood bank or transfusion service shall have methods to limit and detect bacterial contamination in all platelet components."[4] Compliance is required by March, 2004.

Overview of Detection Methods

Detection methods vary in technique and sensitivity. Ideally, a testing system to identify bacterial contamination should be rapid, sensitive, specific, and simple. A rapid assay optimizes prevention of infectious transmission and allows timely issue of products. To optimize identification of as many contaminates as possible, the test should be sensitive and at the same time specific, reducing the number of false-positive results and unnecessarily discarded components. In general, the more rapid the bacteria detection assay, the lower the sensitivity. Simplicity of the method should yield ease of use, implementation, and interpretation.[5]

Appropriate timing of testing is essential to ensure accuracy of the testing results. Unlike viral contamination of blood components, which are detected from a sample obtained at the time of donation, bacterial contamination of blood components generally requires time for the organisms to proliferate before being detectable in a small representative sample from the unit. Therefore, knowledge of the growth characteristics of bacteria in blood components is essential before one considers implementation of a detection strategy. Bacteria can proliferate from low concentrations [<1 colony-forming unit (CFU)/mL] at the time of collection to very high concentrations (>1 × 10^8 CFU/mL) during storage of liquid blood components.[1] Culture studies performed on both Red Blood Cell (RBC) units and platelets have shown that culture on the day of collection invariably misses bacterially contaminated units that would possibly achieve dangerous levels of overgrowth.[6]

Blajchman et al[6] found a contamination rate of 0.02% when 16,290 platelet units were cultured on the day of collection using an automated liquid culture system (Bactec, Becton Dickinson, Cockeysville, MD). However, 2 days later, when the remaining 10,065 units were re-cultured, the contamination rate was 0.07%. Brecher et al studied the growth characteristics of 165 platelet units inoculated on the day of collection with one of the following: *Bacillus cereus, Pseudomonas aeruginosa, Klebsiella pneumoniae, Serratia marcescens, Staphylococcus aureus*, and *Staphylococcus epidermidis.*[7] All examples of *B. cereus, P. aeruginosa, K. pneumoniae, S. marcescens*, and *S. aureus* had concentrations ≥ 10^2 CFU/mL by day 3 following inoculation and by day 4 all units contained ≥ 10^5 CFU/mL. Units contaminated with *S. epidermidis* showed slower and more varied growth. This study suggests that an assay capable of detecting 10^2 CFU/mL on day 3 of storage would detect the vast majority of bacterially contaminated platelet units. Representative growth curves of a variety of bacteria in platelet units are shown in Fig 3-1.

Most commonly implicated in red cell contamination are *Yersinia enterocolitica, Serratia* (*liquifaciens* or *marcescens*), and *Pseudomonas* species as these organisms are capable of growth at 1 to 6 C. It has been demonstrated that the degree of contamination of red cell components is directly related to its storage time. For example, most cases of *Yersinia* contamination occur in blood bags older than 25 days.[8]

Bacterial Culture

BacT/ALERT

Currently available automated liquid media culture systems, such as the BacT/ALERT (bioMérieux), are readily accessible to most large hospital laboratories. The BacT/ALERT automated microbial detection system uses a colorimetric sensor at

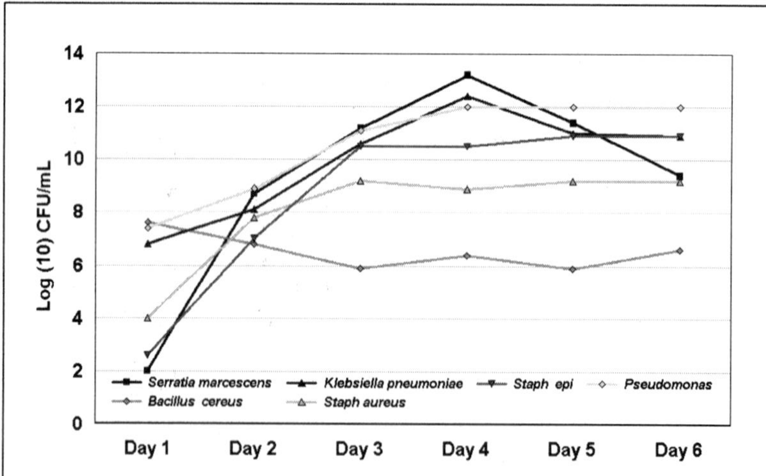

Figure 3-1. Growth curves of six bacteria species (*Serratia marcescens* n = 7, *Klebsiella pneumoniae* n = 21, *Staphylococcus epidermidis* n = 21, *Pseudomonas* species n = 15, *Bacillus cereus* n = 9, and *Staphylococcus aureus* n = 22) in 95 platelet units. All bacteria were inoculated at 10 to 50 CFU/mL on day 0.[7]

the bottom of the culture bottles that changes color in the presence of carbon dioxide produced by bacterial proliferation. The bottles are examined approximately every 10 minutes and the computer software monitors both the rate of change in the colorimetric sensor and the absolute degree of change in the sensor (Fig 3-2).

The sampling of a platelet bag must be performed so as to maintain a sterile, effectively closed system (ie, the bag must not be "spiked"). A variety of sampling bags/sets are commercially available (Fig 3-3). Typically, 3 to 5 mL from the platelet bag are inoculated into culture bottles and incubated on the machine for 5 to 7 days.[9] This system is not completely closed, as a needle is used to inoculate the bottles. If the equipment is not already available in an accessible microbiology laboratory, the initial cost of the equipment is costly. The BacT/ALERT 3D system is approved by the FDA for use with leukocyte-reduced apheresis platelets.[2]

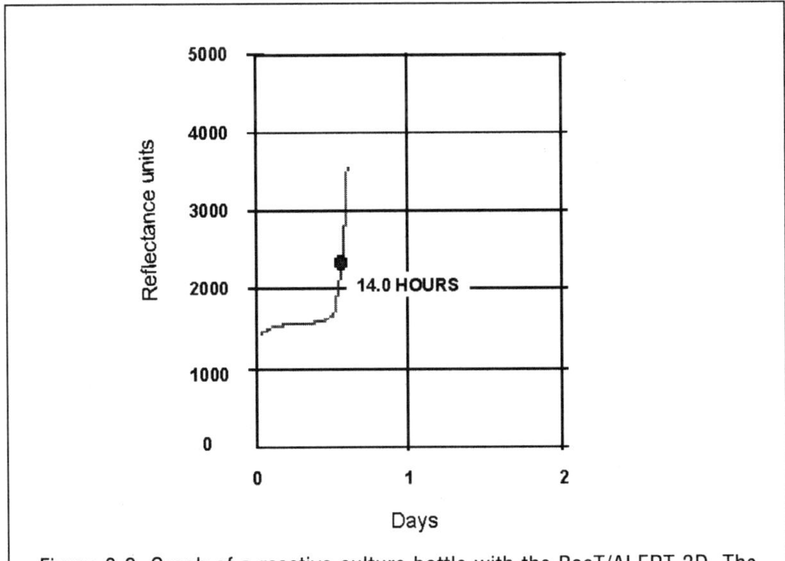

Figure 3-2. Graph of a reactive culture bottle with the BacT/ALERT 3D. The computer software plots the reflectance units of the colorimetric sensor (y-axis) vs time (x-axis).

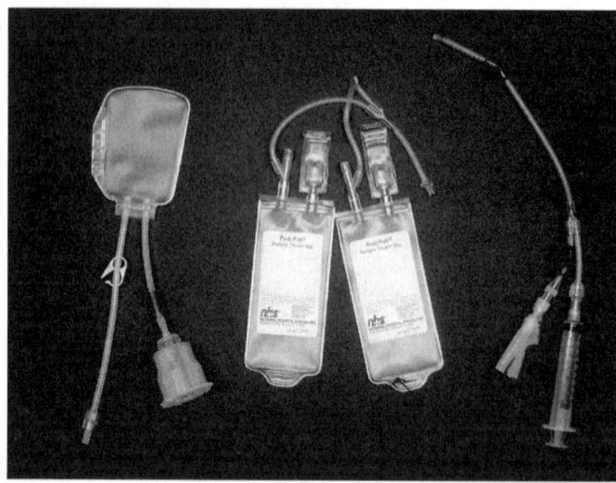

Figure 3-3. Various sampling bags/devices available for platelet bacterial culturing. All bags/devices must be attached using a sterile connection. The bag on the left has an integrated bottle adaptor that contains a sheathed needle. The bags in the middle are pediatric blood bags that contain an integral sample site coupler. The device on the right consists of a syringe and a needle.

The BacT/ALERT has been validated with 14 organisms inoculated into day 2 apheresis platelets (day 0 equals day of collection) at a concentration of 10 CFU/mL and cultured in replicate (Fig 3-4). With the exception of *Propionibacterium acnes* (not shown), which is of questionable clinical significance, all contaminates were detected on average in 9.2 to 25.6 hours.[10,11] Examples of organisms quantitated at ≤ 3 CFU/mL (eg, *B. cereus, S. marcescens, Clostridium perfringens, S. epidermidis, Streptococcus pyogenes*) have been detected within similar time frames.[10,11]

Recently, the implementation and monitoring of the predictive value of a day 2 culture of apheresis platelets have been explored at the University of North Carolina at Chapel Hill (which collects the majority of the platelets transfused) during an 11-month pilot program.[9] The true positive rate for aerobic organisms was 3/2397 (0.13% or 1/799 units) and 4/2397 (0.17% or 1/599 units) for anaerobic organisms. This study de-

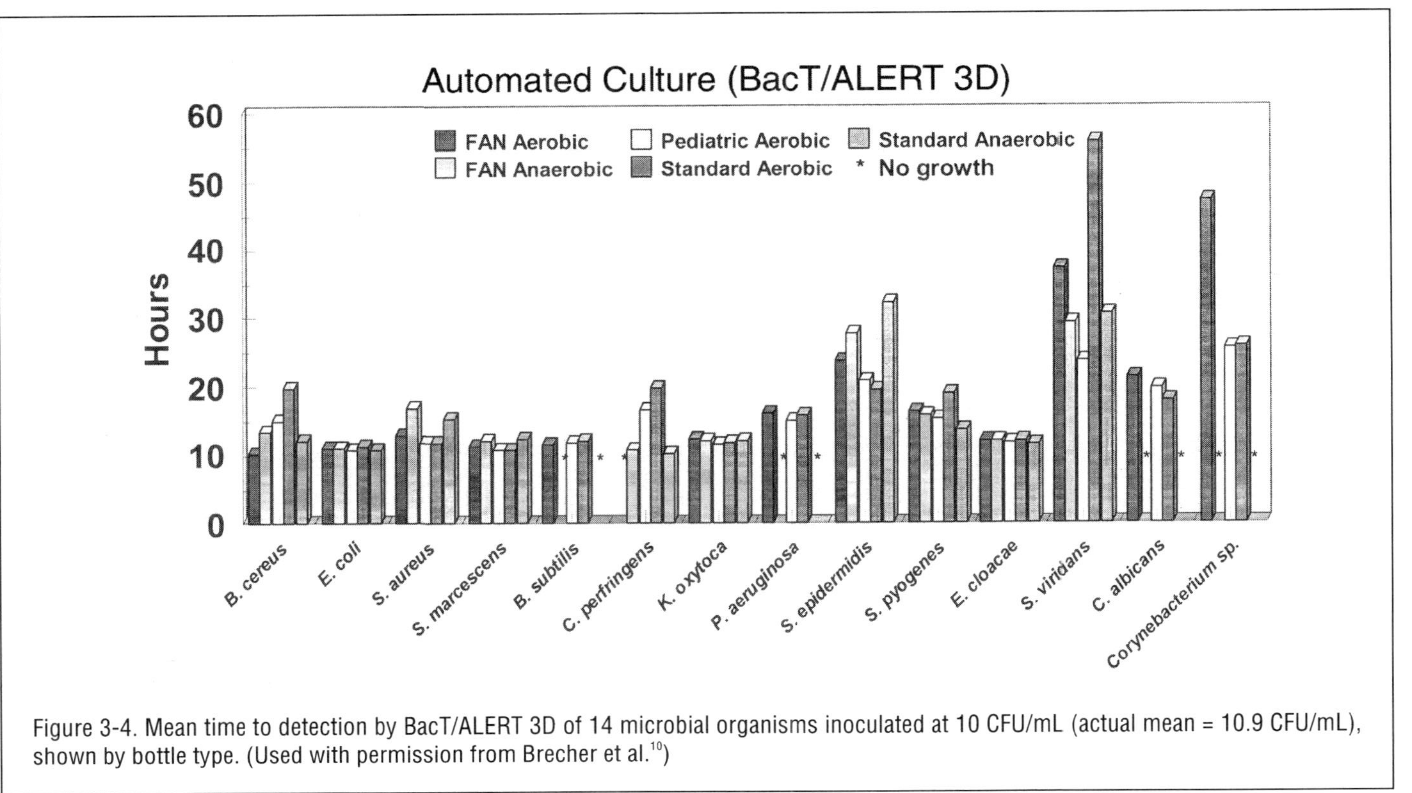

Figure 3-4. Mean time to detection by BacT/ALERT 3D of 14 microbial organisms inoculated at 10 CFU/mL (actual mean = 10.9 CFU/mL), shown by bottle type. (Used with permission from Brecher et al.[10])

tected three platelet bags contaminated with *S. epidermidis* and was able to remove those bags from inventory before patient transfusion. This study's low false-positive rate (due to inadvertent contamination of a bottle or a machine misread) was 2/4794 samplings (0.04% or 1/2397 samplings) or 2/9588 bottles (0.02% or 1/4794 bottles) and may be attributable to the use of a laminar flow hood and the exclusive use of a limited number of research personnel (n = 2).

Pall BDS

A second culture system recently approved by the FDA is the Pall Bacterial Detection System.[2] This method utilizes oxygen concentration to detect microorganisms in leukocyte-reduced apheresis and whole-blood-derived platelet products. Within this effectively closed system, approximately 6 mL of leukocyte-reduced platelet-rich plasma is removed from the component bag and passed through a filter that removes remaining white cells and platelets but allows approximately 50% of bacteria (dependent on organism) with plasma to pass into an incubation bag (Fig 3-5). The bag holds 2 mL and contains sodium polyethanol sulfonate (SPS), which interferes with natural bacterial inhibitors present in blood. The sample bag is then incubated at 35 C for 24 to 30 hours and the oxygen concentration of the bag's headspace is measured with an oximeter. A decrease in the percent oxygen to a level of 19.5% or below is indicative of bacterial growth. In experiments with whole-blood-derived and apheresis platelets inoculated with 10 different bacteria at levels of 100 to 500 CFU/mL at day 1 (100-1200 CFU/mL for apheresis), after 24 hours, 96% of platelet concentrates and 98% of apheresis units tested positive (Table 3-1).[12] Measuring at 30 hours improves sensitivity for the slower growing organism, *S. epidermidis*. Recently published preliminary data report positive results in 80%, 94.2%, and 98.3% of buffy coat platelet concentrates tested at 24, 30, and 48 hours after inoculation with 100 CFU/mL of 12 different organisms.[13]

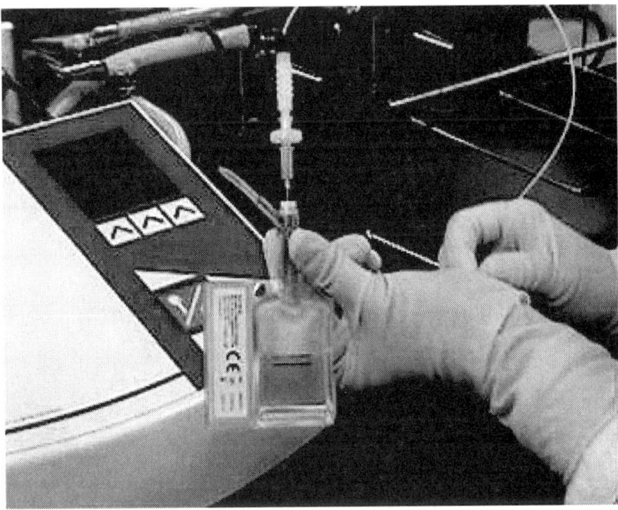

Figure 3-5. The oximeter probe inserted into the sample bag aspirates the headspace air. A pass or fail reading is displayed.

Microscopic Examination

An inexpensive, but less sensitive, detection method is microscopic examination of a stained slide (eg, Gram's stain). Reik and Rubin found in buffy coat smears that Gram's stains were negative at concentrations at or below 1×10^4 CFU/mL, but rare organisms were identified at 4×10^4 CFU/mL.[14] At 1.3×10^6 CFU/mL, 50 to 100 organisms were seen per high power field. Sensitivity and specificity of Gram's stain were reported by one study to be 80% and 99.96% in contaminated platelets aged 1 to 5 days. In 4- to 5-day-old platelets, the sensitivity improved to 100%, with a specificity of 99.93%. True-positive results were associated with bacterial concentrations greater than 10^6 CU/mL.[15] A higher rate of false positives was obtained in a study of 5334 platelet units in which eight positive Gram's stains resulted in only two confirmations by culture.[16]

Use of acridine orange for identification of contamination in platelet components has shown high sensitivity, with one

Table 3-1. Pall BDS Bacterial Detection Data*

Bacteria	Whole-Blood-Derived Platelet Units†	Apheresis Platelet Units†
Staphylococcus aureus	20/20	10/10
Klebsiella pneumoniae	19/20‡	10/10
Serratia marcescens	20/20	10/10
Staphylococcus epidermidis§	19/20§	8/10§
Streptococcus, β-hemoglobin group B§	17/22§	10/10
Salmonella species	20/20	10/10
Bacillus cereus	20/20	10/10
Escherichia coli	20/20	10/10
Enterobacter cloacae	20/20	10/10
Pseudomonas aeruginosa	20/20	10/10

*Modified from the package insert.

†Number detected at 24 hours/number tested; Inoculum: Whole-blood-derived units, 100-500 CFU/mL and Apheresis units,100-1200 CFU/mL.

‡Remaining undetected units tested and detected at 30 hours.

§Remaining undetected unit was not tested at 30 hours.

study detecting bacteria in 100% of platelets with CFUs greater than 10^6 CFU/mL and 83% of platelets at 10^5 to 10^6 CFU/mL.[17] With fluorescent microscopy, acridine orange has been shown to consistently detect bacteria concentrations of 10^4 to 10^5 CFU/mL of *Y. enterocolitica* in RBC products.[18] McCarthy and Senne detected *Escherichia coli* at 1.4×10^4 CFU/mL and *S. aureus* at 8.3×10^3 CFU/mL in broth suspension with acridine orange.[19] Although sensitivity is generally a log greater than with Gram's stain, the process requires use of a fluorescence microscope and acridine orange (a mutagenic compound).

Although not reported or widely implemented, the use of Wright's stain for bacteria detection offers several potential advantages over the use of Gram's stain. Organisms are often easily identified with this stain and less artifact may be present than with Gram's stain. As many hospital laboratories are equipped with automated Wright's stainers, they can provide consistent high quality, reproducible staining. Although all organisms stain blue, initial identification of contamination is a the first priority; classification of gram-negative or -positive status can follow.

Multireagent Strips

Most proliferating bacteria metabolize glucose and produce acid. Thus, diminished glucose and pH levels would be expected in platelet components contaminated with bacteria. Several studies have investigated the use of glucose and pH on multireagent strips (dipsticks) for rapid detection of bacteria in platelet concentrates (PC). One advantage of this process is the rapidity with which results are obtained—30 seconds for glucose and 60 seconds for pH. Overall sensitivity (95%) has been shown to approximate 10^7 CFU per mL, which is similar to the degree of sensitivity of a Gram's stain (10^6 to 10^8 CFU per mL). Wagner and Robinette[20] inoculated PCs with one of seven strains of bacteria, while Burstain et al[21] studied five bacteria species. In some cases, Burstain identified *S. aureus* and *K. pneumoniae* at levels of 10^3 to 10^5 CFU/mL. Recently, Werch et al[22] reported the largest series of prospective surveillance of platelet concentrates screened with reagent strips. Of 3093 PCs, 30 had strips with glucose or pH outside the reference range. Two of these platelets were culture positive for *B. cereus*. Although this less specific screening method prevented two patients from receiving contaminated platelets, it resulted in 9.7 units per 1000 being "wasted."

Anticoagulants and methods of processing are possible sources of variation; therefore, each type of collection requires validation before implementation of such a detection strategy.[20] Measurement of pH can be confusing as pH values are not always reduced in the presence of specific bacteria and may even be elevated. For example, *Klebsiella* species, which metabolize citrate after exhausting the glucose supply, can result in an alkaline bag.[21]

Visual Inspection

Red Blood Cells—Color Change

Kim et al[23] proposed a simple technique for examining the color of RBC units. Darkening of the unit compared to the red cells in the attached sterile tubing segments is indicative of bacteria. This technique has subsequently been confirmed by several authors.[24,25] Contaminated units, when compared to sterile units, become noticeably darker in color 1.5 to 2 weeks after the organism is detected by culture. The darkening of color is due to bacterial proliferation, which causes hemolysis and decreased pO_2. Due to the ease, rapidity, low cost, and noninvasive nature of this testing, detection of contaminated blood units through visual inspection is appealing. However, the sensitivity of the method is considerably lower than other available methods. A recent study found bacterial concentrations in the range of 1.8×10^4 to 1.6×10^9 CFU/mL at the time that RBC units were first identified by visual inspection as potentially contaminated.[26]

Platelets—Swirling

"Swirling" has been described as an alternative visual inspection method for evaluating platelet viability and possible bacterial metabolism. Platelets with discoid morphology (and better viability) reflect light and produce a "swirling" or "streaming" phenomenon, while nondiscoid, spherical platelets do not show this effect. Bacterial metabolism produces a lower pH, leading to a decrease in the "swirling" effect. In one study, platelets ceased to swirl at bacterial levels of 10^7 to 10^8 CFU/mL.[20] Additionally, it has been reported that in some cases, as many as 18% of day 5 platelets may not swirl.[27] Discarding such a high percentage of platelets would be cost prohibitive.

Endotoxin

A cell wall component of gram-negative bacteria, lipopolysaccharide (LPS), is responsible for the symptoms of gram-negative sepsis syndrome. The LPS or endotoxin levels can be measured; however, use in blood component screening is of limited value as it detects only endotoxin-producing organisms. Endotoxin testing is more rapid than culture. Newer quantitative chromogenic testing based upon the use of *Limulus* amebocyte lysate, more sensitive than previous semiquantitative gel-clot assays. Evaluation of endotoxin levels in septic patients has indicated significant binding of LPS to platelets and has suggested that the concentration of LPS in platelet-rich plasma correlates positively with the percentage of LPS platelet binding.[28] Although endotoxin has been shown to bind to platelets by the lipid A portion of the LPS, the impact upon platelet components and clinical significance have not been evaluated.

Endotoxin is also bound to erythrocytes, neutrophils, monocytes, and plasma components. Endotoxin production in RBC units was identified utilizing the *Limulus* amebocyte lysate assay as early as 6 days following inoculation with *Y. enterocolitica,* with the lower limit of bacteria detection in the range of 10^3 CFU/mL.[18]

Another investigator detected endotoxin in RBC units after 21 days of storage, with concentrations at first detection in the range of 10^1 to 10^5 CFU/mL.[8]

In these studies, endotoxin was not detected in 2 units with CFUs/mL in the 10^2 to 10^3 range; one was tested on day 3 and the other on day 14.

Molecular Techniques

Molecular biologic approaches are appealing for the detection of bacterial contamination of blood components because of their high sensitivity and specificity. Probes to a universally conserved bacterial RNA or DNA target or a cocktail of primers and probes to all of the clinically significant bacteria would have to be used to successfully apply this approach. However, several factors potentially limit the direct application of bacterial amplification to blood components. Among the most important of these are bacteria-derived DNA contamination of nucleotide amplification reagents (particularly the bacteria-derived enzymes) and laboratory materials and the presence of bacterial DNA sequences commonly found in human blood.[29,30]

Polymerase Chain Reaction

A study that investigated the use of the polymerase chain reaction (PCR) in the detection of *Y. enterocolitica* in whole blood was able to detect as few as 500 organisms per 100 mL of blood (5×10^3 CFU/mL).[31] Recently, Sen developed a 5′ nuclease TaqMan PCR assay probe based on the nucleotide sequence of the 16S rRNA gene from *Y. enterocolitica*.[32] The TaqMan PCR assay detected as few as six bacteria spiked in 200 microliters (30 CFU/mL) within 2 hours. Another multiplex PCR assay detected 12 to 16 organisms of *Y. enterocolitica, S. liquefaciens, Enterobacter cloacae*, and *K. pneumoniae* in 1 mL of blood.[33]

Bacterial rRNA Probes

The use of a nonamplified chemiluminescence-linked universal bacterial rRNA probe is an alternative approach.[34,35] This method uses an acridinium ester-labeled single-stranded DNA probe complementary to highly conserved bacterial rRNA regions. This technique used for detecting platelet samples contaminated with one of four bacterial species was evaluated by a multicenter trial. All platelet samples with bacterial concentrations of 2.1×10^5 CFU/mL or greater yielded positive results. In the range of 10^4 to 10^5 CFU/mL, 92% of units contaminated with *S. epidermidis* were detected and, in some cases, *S. aureus* was detected at levels as low as 10^2 to 10^3 CFU/mL. The specificity was 100% at thresholds of either 15,000 or 30,000 relative light units when a 0.4-mL platelet sample was used. Chongokolwatana et al[17] reported similar results when comparing the superior performance of the rRNA probe with Gram's and acridine orange stains in detecting platelet contamination at levels of 10^2 to 10^5 CFU/mL.[17]

Microvolume Fluorimetry

The use of fluorescence-labeled antibiotics as probes combined with microvolume fluorimetry is a novel approach for detecting bacterial contamination of blood components. Microvolume fluorimetry is similar to flow cytometry except that the sample remains stationary within a volumetric capillary, and a helium neon laser scans 40 mm of the capillary length. A filter splits two fluorescent signals for low and high wavelength while photomultiplier tubes create a two-color, two-dimensional image of the labeled cells within the capillary (Fig 3-6).[36-39] Antibiotics are potentially ideal molecules for bacterial probes. They have an affinity for bacteria (prokaryotes) over human (eukaryotic) cells, are available in large concentrations, and are inexpensive in comparison with monoclonal antibodies. In one preliminary study, fluorescence-labeled vancomycin was used to detect contamination of platelets with *S. epidermidis* at levels of 2×10^5 CFU/mL.[40]

Peptidoglycan Binding Technology

Preliminary studies of a rapid (25-minute) assay for bacterial contamination detection that employs the proteins and derived peptides that bind to the peptidoglycan component of the bacterial cell wall have been published.[41] Platelets are aspirated through a filter, which captures the bacteria. A biotin label permits the detection of binding activity by standard

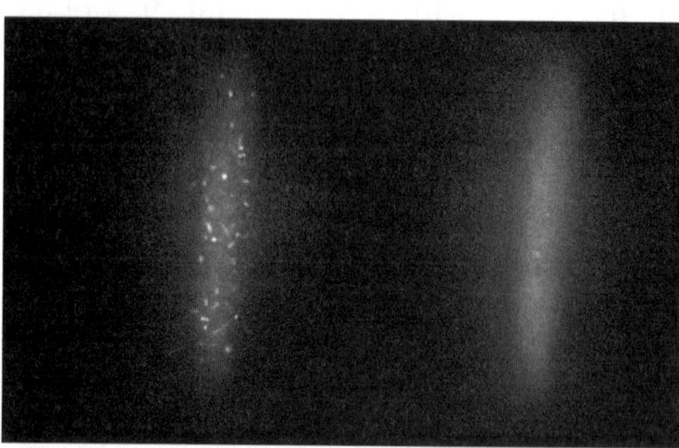

Figure 3-6. Microvolume fluorimetry fluorescent microscopy. Polymyxin-labeled *Serratia marcescens* in capillary tube. Left = Tube containing *S. marcescens.* Right = Sterile tube.

enzymatic means. Eight gram-negative and three gram-positive species of bacteria were spiked into platelet concentrates. All 11 species were detected by the peptidoglycan-binding proteins, and two of four synthetic peptides at densities between 10^3 and 10^4 cells/mL were detected in the concentrate. The other two peptides were inactive and were used as controls. Although this method is quick and also has the potential for use with red cells, to date it has not been validated in external clinical laboratories.[41]

Detection Systems Recently Approved in Europe

Recently, two bacteria detection systems have been approved for use in Europe.

Scansystem

The Scansystem (Hemosystem, Marseille, France) involves a platelet sample that is mixed with a platelet aggregation/DNA labeling solution. After 40 minutes, this mixture is filtered through a membrane that retains the aggregated platelets.[42] The bacteria-laden solution is incubated an additional 20 minutes to enhance fluorescent labeling and is then filtered through a black membrane that retains the bacteria. The black membrane is placed on the instrument. The analyzer, a solid-phase cytometer, uses a laser to detect any fluorescent signal on the membrane; if fluorescence is detected, the user confirms the results using a microscope. Preliminary results show that 100% of the test samples containing bacteria at $\geq 10^3$ CFU/mL were reported as positive (Table 3-2). A preliminary report of the Scansystem detects three gram-positive bacteria species—*S. aureus, S. epidermidis,* and *Streptococcus pyogenes*—within 70 minutes in samples from PCs containing more than 10 CFU/mL.[43] Positive samples require a technologist to perform a microscopic confirmation.

Dielectrophoresis

A second "rapid" method recently approved for use in Europe detects bacteria using dielectrophoresis (Cell Analysis, Slough, United Kingdom). In this application, detection takes advantage of the fact that cells placed in non-uniform electric fields move toward and collect upon electrodes as determined by dielectric properties (conductivity and permittivity) rather than by charge. Platelet concentrates spiked with six organisms at concentrations of 10^1 to 10^6 CFU/mL were studied after 30 minutes of dielectrophoresis by image analysis as the bacteria were released from the electrodes when the electric field was discontinued. Detection levels were from 10^3 CFU/mL to 10^5 CFU/mL.[44]

The Prospect of 7-Day Storage with Detection

The prospect of bacteria detection has raised the possibility of extending the shelf life of platelet components. In 1982, platelet storage was extended from 3 days to 5, then to 7 days in 1983. However, within 3 years after reports of bacterial sepsis followed the transfusion of older units, the FDA returned

Table 3-2. Percentage of Scansystem Positive Results*

Bacteria	n	Bacteria Concentration (CFU/mL)			
		10	**100**	**1000**	**10000**
Gram-positive					
Staphylococcus aureus	42	61%	79%	100%	100%
Staphylococcus epidermidis					
Streptococcus pyogenes					
Streptococcus bovis					
Bacillus cereus					
Gram-negative					
Serratia marcescens	35	84%	90%	100%	100%
Escherichia coli					
Klebsiella pneumoniae					
Pseudomonas aeruginosa					
TOTAL	77	72%	84%	100%	100%

*Modified from the package insert.

the outdate to 5 days.[45] Reports from Europe have described the use of platelet culture on days 1 to 3 of storage to extend the shelf life of platelets to 7 days, thereby reducing the number of outdates.[46-49] Similarly, a recent report from the United States concluded that with the implementation of bacteria screening methods, not only would the extension of storage to 7 days be feasible, but also the additional cost of culturing could be mitigated by the savings obtained from the extension of platelet storage time.[50]

Conclusion

Bacterial contamination is primarily a problem with cellular components in liquid storage. Platelets are of particular concern due to the requirement for storage at room temperature. As a result, efforts to screen for bacterial contamination have focused upon apheresis and whole-blood-derived platelet components. A range of sensitivity and specificity has been reported for the methods presented (Fig 3-7). Among these various detection schemes, three are the most widely implemented: culture, Gram's stain, and multireagent strips. Only two methods, both culture techniques (BacT/ALERT and Pall BDS), have been approved by the FDA in the United States for in-run quality control of platelets. Additional more rapid, but less sensitive, methods are available in Europe. Although recent advances in testing systems and their ability to detect bacteria are improving the safety of the blood supply, the perfect testing system does not exist. Research and development continue in the quest for a screening process that possesses all of the ideal criteria for detection of bacterial contamination—rapidity, sensitivity, specificity, simplicity, and cost-effectiveness.

Acknowledgment

The authors thank James P. AuBuchon, MD, for his collaboration in creating the diagram in Appendix 3-1.

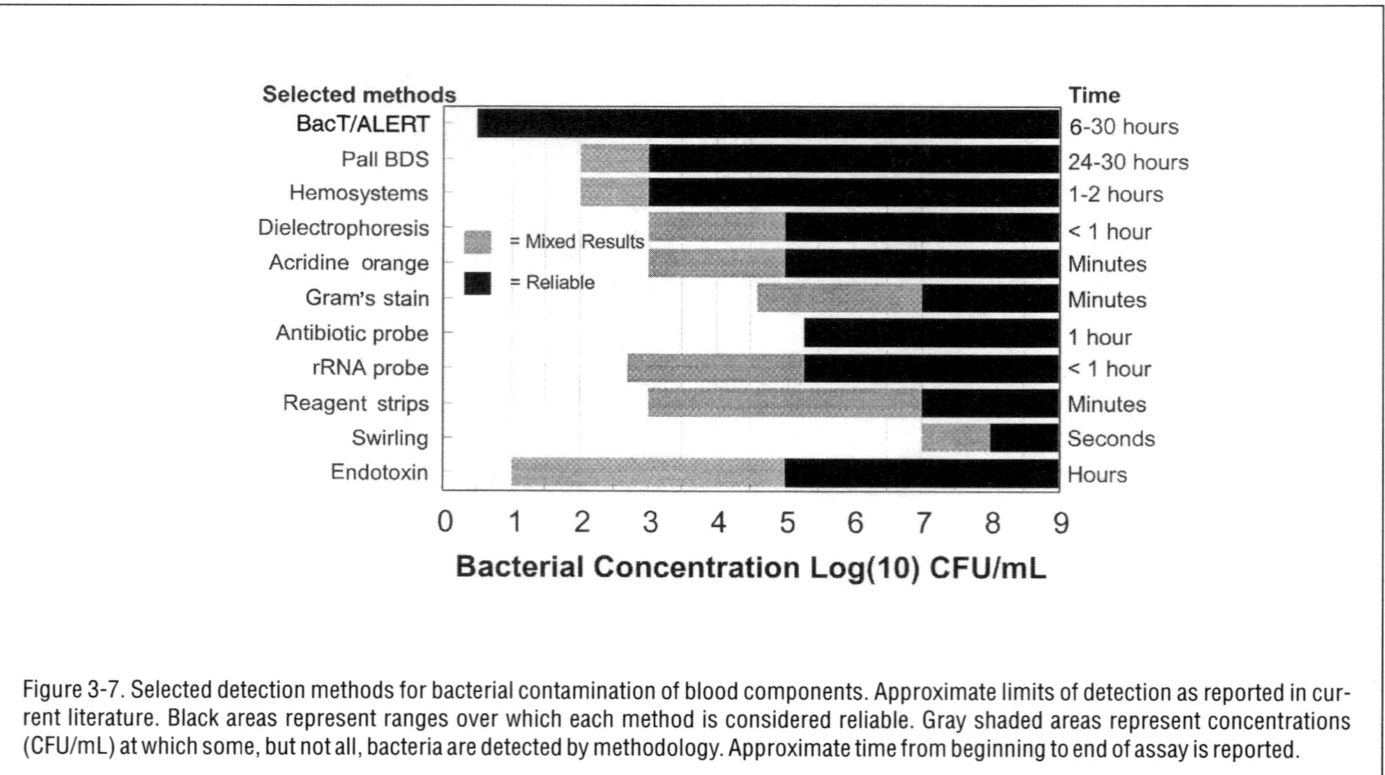

Figure 3-7. Selected detection methods for bacterial contamination of blood components. Approximate limits of detection as reported in current literature. Black areas represent ranges over which each method is considered reliable. Gray shaded areas represent concentrations (CFU/mL) at which some, but not all, bacteria are detected by methodology. Approximate time from beginning to end of assay is reported.

References

1. Goodnough LT, Shander A, Brecher ME. Transfusion medicine: Looking to the future. Lancet 2003;361:161-9.
2. 2002 Biological device application approvals. BacT/ALERT SA culture bottles, 10/10/2002 and Pall bacterial detection system (BDS), 10/22/02. [Available at www.fda.gov/cber/appr2002/2002dev.htm.]
3. Commission on laboratory accreditation, transfusion medicine checklist. TRM.44955 Phase I. Northfield, IL: College of American Pathologists, January 2003. [Available at http://www.cap.org/html/checklist_html/transfusionmedicine_1202.html.]
4. Fridey J, ed. Standards for blood banks and transfusion services. 22nd ed. Bethesda, MD: American Association of Blood Banks, 2003:13.
5. Mitchell K, Brecher M. Approaches to the detection of bacterial contamination in cellular blood products. Transfus Med Rev 1999;13:132-44.
6. Blajchman MA, Ali A, Lyn P, et al. Bacterial surveillance of platelet concentrates: Quantitation of bacterial load (abstract). Transfusion 1997;37(Suppl):74S.
7. Brecher ME, Holland PV, Pineda A, et al. Bacterial growth in inoculated platelets: Implications for bacterial detection and the extension of platelet storage. Transfusion 2000;40:1308-12.
8. Arduino AM, Bland LA, Tipple MA, et al. Growth and endotoxin production of *Yersinia enterocolitica* and *Enterobacter agglomerans* in packed erythrocytes. J Clin Microbiol 1989;27:1483-5.
9. Brecher ME, Hay SN, Rothenberg SJ. Monitoring of apheresis platelet bacterial contamination with an automated liquid culture system: A university experience. Transfusion 2003;43:974-8.
10. Brecher ME, Means N, Jere CS, et al. Evaluation of the BacT/ALERT 3D microbial detection system for platelet bacterial contamination: An analysis of 15 contaminating organisms. Transfusion 2001;41:477-82.
11. Brecher ME, Heath D, Hay S, et al. Evaluation of a new generation culture bottle using the BacT/ALERT 3D microbial detection system on 9 common contaminating organisms found in platelet components. Transfusion 2002;42:774-9.
12. Bacteria detection system for leukocyte-reduced platelet transfusion products—sample set. Pall BDS package insert. East Hills, NY: Pall Corporation, January 2003.
13. McDonald CP, Smith R, Colvin R, et al. Evaluation of the Pall bacterial detection system (BDS). Vox Sang 2002;83(Suppl 2):018.
14. Reik H, Rubin SJ. Evaluation of the buffy-coat smear for rapid detection of bacteremia. JAMA 1981;245:357-9.
15. Yomtovian R, Lazarus HM, Goodnough LT, et al. A prospective microbiologic surveillance program to detect and prevent the transfusion of bacterially contaminated platelets. Transfusion 1993;33:902-9.

16. Barrett BB, Andersen JW, Anderson KC. Strategies for the avoidance of bacterial contamination of blood components. Transfusion 1993;33:228-33.
17. Chongokolwatana V, Morgan M, Feagin JC, et al. Comparison of microscopy and a bacterial DNA probe for detecting bacterially contaminated platelets (abstract). Transfusion 1993;33(Suppl):50S.
18. Kim DM, Brecher ME, Bland LA, et al. Prestorage removal of *Yersinia enterocolitica* from red cells with white cell-reduction filters. Transfusion 1992;32:658-62.
19. McCarthy LR, Senne JE. Evaluation of acridine orange stain for detection of microorganisms in blood cultures. J Clin Microbiol 1980;11:281-5.
20. Wagner SJ, Robinette D. Evaluation of swirling, pH, and glucose tests for the detection of bacterial contamination in platelet concentrates. Transfusion 1996;36:989-93.
21. Burstain JM, Brecher ME, Workman K, et al. Rapid identification of bacterially contaminated platelets using reagent strips: Glucose and pH analysis as markers of bacterial metabolism. Transfusion 1997; 37:255-8.
22. Werch JB, Mhawech P, Stager CE, et al. Detecting bacteria in platelet concentrates by use of reagent strips. Transfusion 2002;42:1027-31.
23. Kim DM, Brecher ME, Bland LA, et al. Visual identification of bacterially contaminated red cells. Transfusion 1992;32:221-5.
24. Franzin L, Gioannini P. Growth of *Yersinia* species in artificially contaminated blood bags. Transfusion 1992;32:673-6.
25. Bradley RM, Gander RM, Patel SK, et al. Inhibitory effect of $0^{\circ}C$ storage on the proliferation of *Yersinia enterocolitica* in donated blood. Transfusion 1992;37:691-5.
26. Pickard C, Herschel L, Seery P, et al. Visual identification of bacterially contaminated red blood cells (abstract). Transfusion 1998;38(Suppl): 12S.
27. Bertolini F, Murphy S. A multicenter evaluation of reproducibility of swirling in platelet concentrates. Transfusion 1994;34:796-801.
28. Salden HJM, Bert MB. Endotoxin binding to platelets in blood from patients with a sepsis syndrome. Clin Chem 1994;40:1575-9.
29. Nikkari S, McLaughin IJ, Bi W, et al. Does blood of healthy subjects contain bacterial ribosomal DNA? J Clin Microbiol 2001;39(5):1956-9.
30. Fredricks DN, Relman DA. Improved amplification of microbial DNA from blood cultures by removal of the PCR inhibitor sodium polyanetholesulfonate. J Clin Microbiol 1998;36(10):2810-6.
31. Feng P, Keasler SP, Hill WE. Direct identification of *Yersinia enterocolitica* in blood by polymerase chain reaction amplification. Transfusion 1992;32:850-4.
32. Sen K. Rapid identification of *Yersinia enterocolitica* in blood by the 5′ nuclease PCR assay. J Clin Microbiol 2000;38:1953-8.
33. Sen K, Asher DM. Multiplex PCR for detection of *Enterobacteriaceae* in blood. Transfusion 2001;41:1356-64.
34. Brecher ME, Hogan JJ, Boothe G, et al. The use of a chemiluminescence-linked universal bacterial ribosomal RNA gene probe and blood

gas analysis for the rapid detection of bacterial contamination in white cell reduced and nonreduced platelets. Transfusion 1993;33:450-7.
35. Brecher ME, Hogan JJ, Boothe G, et al. Platelet bacterial contamination and the use of a chemiluminescence-linked universal bacterial ribosomal RNA gene probe. Transfusion 1994;34:750-5.
36. Dietz L, Debrow RS, Manian BS, et al. Volumetric capillary cytometry—a new method for absolute cell enumeration. Cytometry 1996;23: 177-86.
37. Lee LG, Woo SL, Head DF, et al. Near-IR dyes in three-color volumetric capillary cytometry: Cell analysis with 633- and 785-nm laser excitation. Cytometry 1995;21:120-8.
38. Dzik WH. A general method for concentrating blood samples in preparation for counting very low numbers of white cells. Transfusion 1997;37:277-83.
39. Adams MR, Johnson DK, Busch MP, et al. Automatic volumetric capillary cytometry for counting white cells in white cell-reduced plateletpheresis components. Transfusion 1997;37:29-37.
40. Brecher ME, Wong ECC, Chen SE, et al. Antibiotic linked probes and microvolume fluorimetry for the rapid detection of bacterial contamination in platelet products. Transfusion 2000;40:411-3.
41. Kagan D, Levin AE. Rapid assay for bacterial contamination of platelets (abstract). Transfusion 2001;41(Suppl):34S.
42. Scansystem^{TM} platelet kit package insert. Marseille, France: Hemosystems, January 2003.
43. Morel P, Deschaseaux M, Bertrand X, et al. Detection of bacterial contamination in platelet concentrates using Scansystem: First results (abstract). Transfusion 2002;42(Suppl):40S.
44. McDonald CP, Smith R, Colvin J, et al. Evaluation of a novel dielectrophoresis system for the rapid detection of bacteria in platelet concentrates (abstract). Transfusion 2001;41(Suppl):34S.
45. Yomtovian R. Bacterial contamination—an overview of key issues. Presented at the FDA/CBER Workshop on Safety and Efficacy of Methods for Reducing Pathogens in Cellular Blood Products Used in Transfusion, Bethesda, MD, August 7-8, 2002. [Available at http://www.fda.gov/cber/minutes/workshop-min.htm.]
46. Ollgaard M, Albjerg I, Georgen J. Monitoring of bacterial growth in platelet concentrates: One year's experience with the BacT/ALERT system. Vox Sang 1998;74(Suppl 1):1126.
47. Vuetic D, Taseki J, Balint B, et al. The use of BacT/ALERT system for bacterial screening in platelet concentrates. Vox Sang 2000;78(Suppl 1):P371.
48. Laan E, Tros C. Improved safety and extended shelf-life of leuco-depleted platelet concentrates by automated bacterial screening (abstract). Transfusion 1999;39(Suppl):5S.
49. McDonald CP, Roy A, Lowe P, et al. The first experience in the United Kingdom of the bacteriological screening of platelets to increase shelf life to 7 days. Vox Sang 2000;78(Suppl):P375.

50. Dumont LJ, AuBuchon JP, Whitey P, et al. Seven-day storage of single-donor platelets: Recovery and survival in an autologous transfusion study. Transfusion 2002;42:847-54.

Appendix 3-1. Example of a Bacteria Detection Algorithm

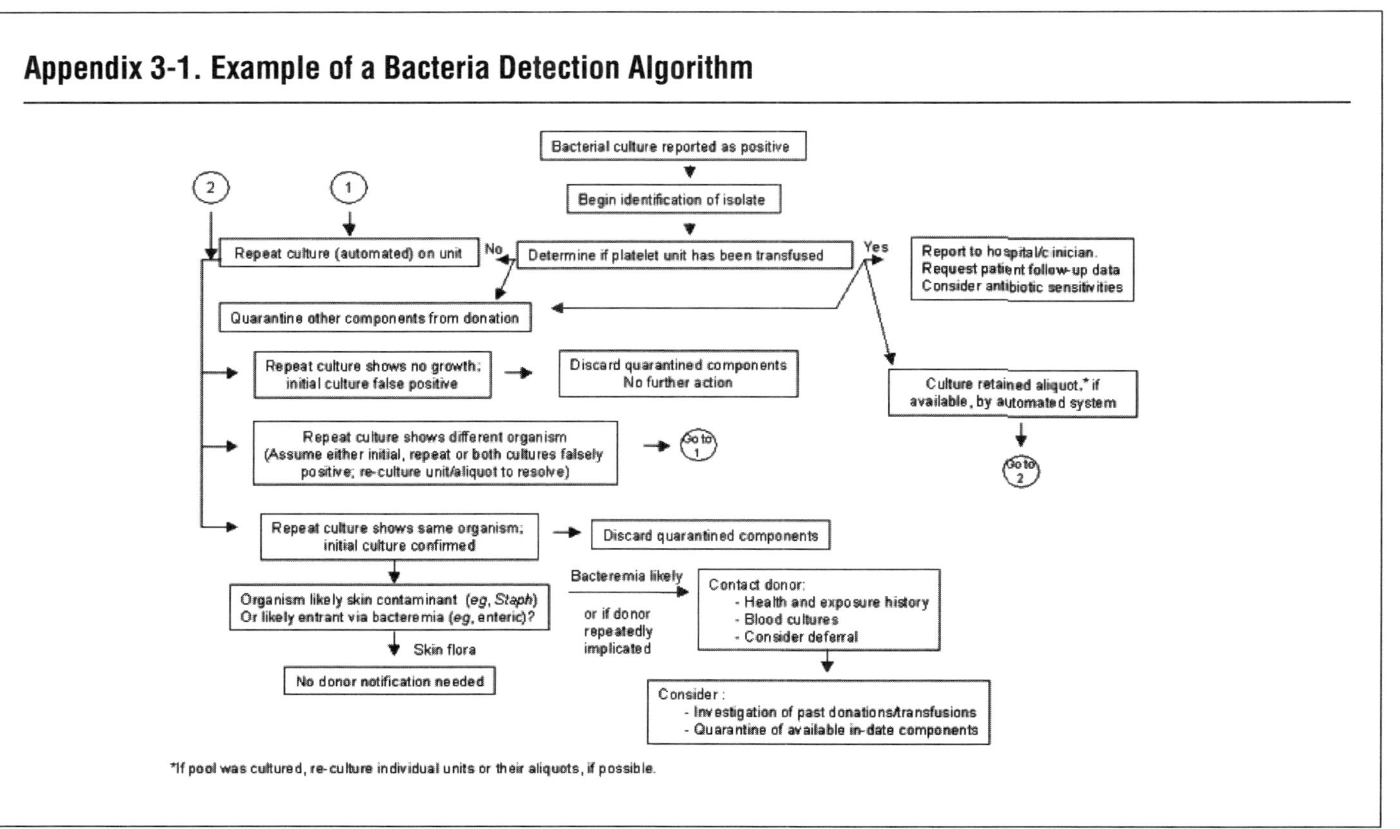

In: Brecher ME, ed.
Bacterial and Parasitic Contamination of Blood Components
Bethesda, MD: AABB Press, 2003

4

Implementation of a Screening System for Bacteria Detection

DIRK DE KORTE, PHD

SINCE THE IMPLEMENTATION OF PROGRAMS for reducing the contamination of the blood supply by blood-borne viruses, transfusion-transmitted bacterial infections (TTBIs) have become one of the major hazards of blood transfusion. Sazama[1] estimated that 10% of blood transfusion-associated deaths are caused by bacterial contamination of the transfused component. The exact prevalence of bacterial contamination of blood components is

Dirk de Korte, PhD, Head of Laboratory for Blood Transfusion Technology, Sanquin Research at CLB, Amsterdam, The Netherlands

unknown, but it can be estimated at the level of 0.4% for apheresis Red Blood Cells (RBCs) and apheresis Platelets and up to 2% for pooled Platelets derived from whole blood donations.[2] For whole blood donations, it has been shown that 0.34% of whole blood units were contaminated with bacteria.[3] That study evaluated a large number of tested units, resulting in a narrow 95% CI of 0.27% to 0.44%.

The incidence of hepatitis C virus (HCV) and human immunodeficiency virus (HIV) infection through blood donation in Western Europe and the United States, after the introduction of nucleic acid amplification testing (NAT), is estimated to range from 0.5 to 1 per 1×10^6 units,[4] much lower than the prevalence of bacterial contamination.[2,5,6] The risk that a Platelet unit will be contaminated with bacteria is much higher than that of viral contamination. Although only a portion of these contaminated blood components results in clinically recognized TTBI in a recipient, the frequency of such infection is considerable. Reliable data on the frequency of TTBI are still rare and highly variable, ranging from 1 per 4000 to 1 per 100,000, also depending on the platelet source (apheresis or whole-blood-derived).[7-10] Because of the lack of precise criteria for TTBI and the fact that clinicians are not always alert for TTBI in the case of transfusion complications, transmission of bacteria by transfusion is underestimated, and reports in the literature are acknowledged to be "the tip of the iceberg."

Increased attention has been given to the prevention of possible contamination during the collection (ie, by disinfection[11-13] or diversion[14-16]) and preparation stages (ie, closed systems, use of sterile connection devices) of blood components.

Another approach receiving much attention is detection of the bacteria in blood components before issuing, either as in-run quality control or as a prerequisite for release of the component.[17-19] Because platelets are generally considered to be the blood component having the highest risk for bacterial contamination, most efforts are focused on platelets. In an indirect way, this increases the microbiologic safety of red cell components. If a Platelet unit prepared from whole blood tests positive for bacterial contamination, in most cases, the related RBC unit can be prevented from being used for transfusion. In some European countries, 100% screening of platelet concentrates has been introduced (obligatory in Belgium and The Netherlands) to prevent as much as possible the introduction of contaminated units in the transfusion chain.

This chapter addresses some practical aspects of implementing a 100% bacterial screening program for platelet concentrates, including:

- Starting up the implementation.
- Information to blood banks and hospitals (producers and consumers).
- Detection system.
- Standardization.
- Inoculation: method, size, and time of sampling.
- Platelet release protocol.
- Policy for related products.
- Follow-up in clinic.
- Prolonged platelet storage.
- Cost-effectiveness.

Starting up the Implementation

Before any measure to improve the safety of blood transfusion with respect to bacterial contamination can be implemented, accurate information on the frequency of bacterial contamination is needed. This frequency depends on many factors, such as methods used for production, storage time, donor population, climate, etc. Thus, it is important to have an up-to-date review of the current situation focused on the blood supply chain in the area or country in which implementation is desired. During this survey period, other measures to reduce the risk of bacterial contamination should also be reviewed, such as 1) improvement of donor skin preparation and/or disinfection, 2) diversion of the first volume of blood collected or 3) the introduction of a pathogen inactivation method.

In The Netherlands, a report was written by an advisory committee for the Medical Advisory Board of the Blood Supply Foundation. This report addressed the status of what was known about bacterial contamination of blood components, methods for prevention, methods for detection, consequences for related products, etc. This report resulted in a recommendation to introduce, as a first measure, 100% bacterial screening, using a culturing method.

This recommendation was adopted by the Ministry of Health and resulted in a Working Party for the Implementation of Bacterial Screening. This Working Party was responsible for the practical aspects of implementation, whereas the Medical Advisory Board was responsible for a national guideline that contained minimum requirements for the blood centers on performing the screening. Such a guideline should contain requirements for a culture system, a sampling and inoculation procedure, a release procedure, a process for managing positive results from the culture system, a method for handling related components (RBCs and plasma), and a means for determining when donor counseling is required. A hemovigilance system should be in place or started in parallel with the implementation of bacterial screening.

The Working Party was responsible for education of the field and for setting up the framework for the practical implementation of the screening. Although each blood center remains responsible for the final implementation, the Working Party appeared to be very effective in supplying standards for the different aspects of implementation, such as the introduction of culture systems in blood bank practice, and providing standard operating procedures for sampling, release, and recall. The Working Party also took care of a nationwide contract with the manufacturer of culture systems and culture bottles, who provided devices, service, and back-up as well.

Information to Blood Banks and Hospitals

Before a system for bacterial screening of blood components is implemented, either on a small scale (one or more blood centers with affiliated hospitals) or on a large scale (nationwide), there should be consensus on the approach. All parties involved should be willing to implement an additional measure—one with the potential for a heavy workload, a complicated recall process, and complex look-back procedures. Therefore, much attention should be given to the education of both producers (blood bank personnel) and consumers (hospital personnel) on the additional screening test. Both basic microbiology and more specific facts on microbiologic contamination of blood components should be incorporated in these educational sessions.

Because several departments of the blood bank are involved (donor selection, blood collection, blood processing, and blood issuing), the education should be broad, to increase awareness of microbiologic contamination during the whole transfusion chain, from donor to patient. In the blood bank, this should start with donor selection, including a recommendation to ask donors to notify the blood bank if they develop symptoms of possible bacteremia in the week following blood donation.[20] Subsequently, attention should be given to donor skin preparation; phlebotomy; and the processing, storage, and issuing of the components. It might be worthwhile to provide general training on risk analysis to responsible blood bank personnel, with microbiologic hazards as a study case, so that all employees understand where contamination can occur.

The so-called Failure Mode Effect and Criticality Analysis (FMECA) can be helpful in this training. In this model all possible causes for failure are analyzed per sub-process and subsequently scored for frequency of the cause (1 - 10 from low to high), chance of detection and prevention (1 - 10 from high to low), and severity of the consequences (1 - 10 from negligible to false result). Multiplication of the scores results in a total score per possible failure cause, giving an indication of the relative risk of that part of the process. Once the results for all process steps are sorted, the high-risk steps in the process can be identified. Priority can be given to preventive measures and/or adaptations of the high-risk steps to lower the overall risk in the most effective way.

For hospitals, one of the goals should be to improve recognition of TTBI (although the overall goal is to prevent TTBI) because it is generally known that this is underreported. Another goal is to explain how bacterial screening is different from standard screening tests for other infectious diseases. In the case of a "negative to date" screening system (see below), the hospital may receive a blood component that is still under investigation. The hospital may even receive the message "culture positive after release from the blood bank." This is unlike the more familiar situation with viral testing, which must be completed before release of the unit. Therefore, clinicians should know how to deal with such messages, not only with respect to the tested component, but also with respect to related components. They should know what the risk of TTBI is for patients in case of positive results in the culture bottle. In other words, clinicians should know the predictive value of both a positive and a "negative to date" flag in the screening system used.

Detection System

The choice for a detection system is based on sensitivity, specificity, and speed of detection. In general, the more rapid a detection method is, the lower its sensitivity and/or specificity. Culturing systems are very sensitive but may require several days to detect a positive unit. With respect to implementation in routine use, other factors are important, such as the degree of automation, simplicity to incorporate in standard practice, reliability, etc. For screening purposes, the logical choice is still a culturing system because other methods based on immediate detection of relatively high levels of microorganisms—such as a polymerase chain reaction (PCR),[21] fluorescence using antibiotic-labeled[22] or bacterial ribosomal RNA gene probes,[23] or automated microscopy in combination with a fluorescent DNA-probe[24]—are still in the development phase. All of these systems are open to question with respect to sensitivity (which should be about 10^2-10^3 CFU/mL or lower, depending on the moment of application), specificity, and practical application, and they must be capable of detecting the broad spectrum of possible species found in blood components.

With respect to culturing systems, there is a choice between the semiautomatic culturing system BacT/ALERT (bioMérieux, Durham, NC), based on the measurement of carbon dioxide production,[25] and the recently introduced nonautomated Bacterial Detection System (BDS, Pall Corporation, East Hills, NY), based on the measurement of oxygen consumption.[26] With large numbers of units to be tested, the BacT/ ALERT is helpful because it is a semiautomated system, requiring fewer manual steps. This system has the potential for a complex computer interface with a blood bank computer system. Even so, the throughput with the BacT/ALERT system is limited: one has to fill culture bottles and load the culture bottles in an incubator, using barcodes to identify and link the culture bottles with the unit tested.

A culturing system in use for bacterial screening of blood components should be equipped with alarm systems that alert personnel of a malfunction 24 hours per day, 7 days per week. Both the culturing and the alarm system should be coupled to an emergency power supply, and there should be an adequate back-up system in case of a prolonged malfunction or other interruption in service.

Standardization

Standardization in screening tests will help ensure comparable safety levels in different blood centers. The inoculation method should be standardized because the time of sampling, the volume, and the conditions during inoculation are crucial for the results. If it is not possible to use exactly the same method for bacterial screening, at least the systems used should be comparable, especially with respect to sensitivity and specificity. There should be agreement on the definition of such terms as confirmation, false-positive, and false-negative.

Also, standard methods and nomenclature for differentiation of bacteria should be used. In The Netherlands, a positive flag in the culture system is called "confirmed" if a bacterium could be subcultured from the culture bottle. This is different from the definition of "confirmed" in some other studies, for example, those by Blajchman et al[6] or Castro and Bueno,[27] in which a case is called "confirmed" only if the same bacterium was isolated from both the culture bottle and the original product tested (or one of the related products). In The Netherlands, the different definition described above was chosen because a limited number of Platelet units were expected to be available for reconfirmation cultures. Furthermore, it was known from other studies that under the conditions used for inoculation (aseptic transfer in a laminar flow with minimal handling), the contamination was less than 0.05% (0 positives in 2000 aseptic transfers[3]).

Therefore, if a subculture can be obtained from a positive screening culture, a sample is called true-positive (this will include some secondary contaminations introduced by the sampling process). If not, it is concluded that the detection system has detected a false-positive signal (failure of the system) or that it was not possible to subculture the bacterium in the culture bottle with the standard procedure used. In the Dutch experience, 93% of the positively flagged bottles resulted in growth in a subculture from the bottles. This figure is very similar to that reported by Schelstraete et al[19] for the Belgian screening results. An indication that this is not merely system failure is the fact that in 16% of the cases with negative subcultures from positively flagged Platelet units, it was possible to isolate a bacterium from one of the related RBC units. The definition of a false-negative result is that despite a negative signal in the culturing system, the unit is found to be positive upon release or during storage. A false-negative result can be due to failure of the system or inadequate numbers of bacteria in the inoculum to grow in the culture bottle, whereas during storage, the few bacteria present in the unit proliferated to levels enabling detection in a later stage.

Inoculation: Method, Size, and Time of Sampling

Method of Inoculation

To limit positive results caused by contamination during the inoculation process as much as possible, the sampling and subsequent inoculation procedure should have a limited number of aseptic steps to be performed. Preference should be given to a sample pouch already coupled to the platelet storage container, which can be filled at the desired moment. In Europe, where most of the Platelet units are prepared from pooled buffy coats, several manufacturers supply complete sets ready for use, consisting of a pooling set, a leukocyte reduction filter, and a platelet storage container with a sampling pouch. With a sterile connection device, the whole product can be manufactured in a closed system, including the sampling for bacterial culture and quality control. Also, for apheresis platelets, containers with an integrated sampling pouch are available.

The sampling pouch can be equipped with a needle or an adapter for aseptic fill of the culture bottles, preferably performed in a laminar flow cabinet. The use of an adapter minimizes the risk of a needlestick during processing manipulations (including centrifugation). However, inoculation with use of an adapter increases the risk for contamination compared with the use of a needle. In practice, this type of positive result (not included in the definition of false positives stated previously because a bacterium will be subcultured from the positively flagged bottle) can be very low, providing adequate (microbiologic) hygienic measures are taken during inoculation. However, it is very hard to distinguish between this type of positive case and positive cases where no positive culture can be achieved from the unit itself upon resampling and subsequent culturing (see also the last paragraph of Time of Sampling and Inoculation).

Size of the Inoculum

Most bacteria are not equally distributed throughout a blood component. Therefore, especially at the relatively low levels to be expected in contaminated platelets early during storage (within 24 hours after whole blood collection), the sample volume should be relatively large to pick up enough microorganisms to induce a positive culture (1 - 10 CFU for the bioMérieux system[25]). The sensitivity will also be increased with the use of two culture bottles. With the use of both an aerobic and an anaerobic bottle, nearly all types of microorganisms will be detected at a very low level in the original inoculum. In spiking studies, most microorganisms are detected very effectively by either aerobic or anaerobic bottles.[25,28,29] However, the use of an anaerobic bottle will detect some strictly anaerobic bacteria that show little or no growth in the aerobic bottle. It is questionable if the combination of an aerobic and an anaerobic bottle will detect any more aerobic bacteria than will two aerobic bottles (especially a clinically relevant organism that can cause a bacterial infection after transfusion). On the basis of the Dutch experience, it seems reasonable to assume that with the combination of a large-volume inoculum (mean, 7.5 mL per bottle) and the use of both an aerobic and an anaerobic bottle, the screening system is detecting microorganisms at the lower level of the detection limit for the culturing system. In the Dutch experience, only 25 of the 474 Platelet units with a positive signal in the culturing system flagged positive for both bottles (with one case of two different bacteria isolated, indicating a contamination during inoculation). This supports the use of two bottles instead of one. Table 4-1 illustrates that different bacteria species are detected adequately by either aerobic or anaerobic culture bottles.

Time of Sampling and Inoculation

With respect to the inoculation moment, there are two possibilities: the sample is inoculated immediately after production or the sample is inoculated after the Platelet unit has been stored for 1 or 2 days. The optimal moment might differ with the component under investigation, with a difference between apheresis platelets and platelets prepared from whole blood

Table 4-1. Positive Signal in Aerobic or Anaerobic Bottle*

	Aerobic	Anaerobic	Total[†]
Staphylococcus species (coagulase-negative)	88	70	148
Bacillus species	17	11	23
Corynebacterium species	10	8	18
All positive cases	171	328	474

*Based on screening results in The Netherlands during 2002 with the bio-Mérieux system.

[†]Totals reflect overlap.

donations. For inoculation immediately after production, the sensitivity of the detection system should be higher than that in a system used for later inoculation. In the latter case, the level of microorganisms in a contaminated unit will already be higher at the moment of inoculation, due to the favorable conditions for bacterial growth in platelets during storage. In a large study, Blajchman et al[6] showed the frequency of false-negative results to be very high in whole-blood-derived platelets. Over 16,000 units were cultured on day 1; 10,065 of these units were also cultured at day 3. All true-positive cultures from day 1 were also positive on day 3. However, the true-positive prevalence was 25 per 100,000 on day 1 and 70 per 100,000 on day 3. Because Blajchman et al used a sample of about 2 mL and only one culture bottle (aerobic), the sensitivity in that study was much lower than in the screening system adopted in The Netherlands. When the Dutch data are adjusted for the number of units in a pooled product, the contamination rate is about 1 true positive per 700 Platelet units (with the same microorganism isolated from the original product).

In contrast, Blajchman et al[6] reported 1 per 4000 at day 1 and 1 per 1400 at day 3. Besides the difference in sensitivity, practice in Europe and the United States/Canada differs in the length of hold times. In Canada and the United States, fewer than 8 hours elapse between whole blood collection and the production of a platelet component, whereas in Europe, there is generally a period of 16 to 24 hours between whole blood collection and component preparation.

A Dutch study[30] with a method similar to the current screening used with whole-blood-derived platelets from pooled buffy coats showed a much more probable frequency of false-negative results (defined as the initial sample taken 2 hours after production being negative, but at repeated sampling after 2 to 4 days found positive). With a total of 2100 Platelet units studied, Laport et al[30] found two samples to be positive when tested after 2 to 4 days, whereas samples from the same unit were negative when sampled 2 hours after pooling on day 0, leading to a false-negative rate of about 0.1%.

When the figures of Blajchman et al[6] showing that two thirds of platelets containing bacteria would not have been detected by cultures at day 1 are extrapolated to the results of the screening system in The Netherlands, an improbable number of more than 1000 contaminated units per year would have been missed. If this was true, there should have been several reports of TTBI during that period, due to the increased awareness on bacterial contamination of blood products. Extrapolation of the figures of Laport et al[30] result in about 50 contaminated units per year that would be missed in the Dutch screening—a number that seems much more likely. With the assumptions that about 40 of these units would be released (many of them before the level of bacteria is harmful to the recipient) and that about 1 in 20 contaminated units will lead to TTBI, one would expect only an incidental case of TTBI.

In summary, for pooled platelets from buffy coats, sampling and inoculation immediately following production (which means about 16 to 24 hours after collection of the whole blood) seem to be the right choice. In a system with an integrated sampling pouch, the sampling is easily integrated with the standard production, with the advantage that the sample can also be used for 100% quality control of the platelet count and/or leukocyte and red cell content. For apheresis platelets, or for whole- blood-derived platelets lacking a long period between whole blood collection and component preparation, it might be advisable to wait some time before inoculation, to allow some proliferation of bacteria present in the component. Also, for this type of component, the use of an integrated sampling pouch is encouraged, allowing easy sampling at the desired moment, with a minimum of aseptic handling to inoculate the culture bottle.

Besides the discussion on false-negative results, another argument for delayed sampling is the so-called self-sterilization. This means that units initially flagged as positive are negative upon repeated sampling after some days of storage. This might be due to killing of the bacteria by complement or other constituents or by an inability of the bacteria introduced by the phlebotomy process to grow in a plasma environment. In some studies, the percentage of units showing this phenomenon is quite high, varying from 37% up to 90%.[20,27,31] In the Dutch experience, it was found to be the case in 37% of initially positive units, whereas in 63% of the repeatedly sampled units, the same microorganism could be isolated—a number that is identical to the number reported for Belgium,[31] using a similar screening approach as in The Netherlands. As stated before, it is very unlikely that such a high percentage is the result of positives caused by secondary contamination during the inoculation process and/or false positives due to failure of the system.

Platelet Release Protocol

When a choice has been made for a screening method for bacterial contamination, there are roughly two possibilities: release of products as "negative to date" or release after a specified quarantine period. Release as "negative to date" means that it is checked to determine whether the component is in culture and whether at the moment of release the unit has tested negative for bacterial contamination. Release after a quarantine period means that the component has been in culture for a minimal time, allowing a positive signal for the most harmful contaminations (fast-growing organisms with a relatively high initial CFU/mL). However, the chance that the culture is positive after 48 hours is relatively high. Because of the short shelf-life of platelets, a quarantine period is practical only if the shelf-life can be prolonged from 5 to 7 days. A quarantine period of 48 hours and a shelf-life of 5 days would mean that there are only about 56 hours left for release because 16 hours will have expired already between collecting whole blood and finalizing the production of a Platelet unit from pooled buffy coats. In order to prolong shelf life, it has to be determined—by in-vitro quality and in-vivo recovery and survival studies—that platelets stored for 7 days are as effective as those stored for 4 to 5 days (see Prolonged Platelet Storage).

From the results of 1 year of screening in The Netherlands, it appears that a quarantine period of 2 days would have prevented 43% (211 units) of the positively flagged units from being released. Quarantine would have been able to prevent the release of more than 90% of units contaminated with the more dangerous bacteria species with respect to TTBI, such as gram-negative bacteria, *Bacillus cereus,* and *Staphylococcus aureus.* When the slow-growing anaerobic bacteria, such as *Propionibacterium* and *Corynebacterium* species, are excluded from this analysis (because they are believed to be of less significance for the problem of TTBI), 65% of positively flagged Platelet units (184 out of 284 units) would have been prevented from being transfused with a quarantine period of 2 days. However, even without a quarantine period, in the Dutch practice, about 90% of the units identified as positive within 2 days remained in the inventory of the blood bank, including the majority of those contaminated with the more dangerous bacteria as described earlier. Most of the units that were already released became positive after 2 or more days of culturing (mean 5.2 days; 93% >2 days) and were mainly found to be contaminated with *Propionibacterium* species. The majority of these units were already transfused; however, no complaints were observed related to transfusion of such units. Therefore, it can be concluded that a screening system based upon release as "negative to date" is successful in preventing seriously contaminated Platelet units from entering the transfusion chain, a similar conclusion reported for Belgium.[31]

Policy for Related Products

In combination with 100% screening of platelets, there should be a system in place for the related products. With platelet products derived from whole blood donations, related components to consider include both plasma and RBC units.

Plasma related to a confirmed-positive Platelet unit should not be used as Fresh Frozen Plasma for transfusion. Although the chance that a bacterium survives frozen storage is minimal, there have been reports of contaminated plasma units.[5] Plasma that is to be pooled and further processed into plasma derivatives will likely have an additional risk of bacterial contamination due to the pooling process. However, overall contamination is less of a concern due to the pathogen reduction steps that are used in preparing such products.

Upon a positive signal in the screening of a platelet component, the related RBCs should be quarantined immediately and, if already released, a recall procedure should be started. If the Platelet unit has been produced from pooled buffy coats, there are generally five related RBC units. It should be clear to the hospital transfusion service that there is a chance that a contaminated RBC unit has been delivered (because it is expected that only one of the donations will be contaminated, the chance is 20%). Because of the much longer shelf-life for RBCs compared with platelet components, usually, the number of RBC units already released will not be high. In the Dutch experience during 2002, a recall was necessary for 18% of the related RBC units (n = 383) and because RBCs are often in stock in the hospital, this recall was successful for 271 of these units (71%). This is in contrast with Platelet units, which were successfully recalled in only 16% of the cases, probably because they are usually released for immediate use. If hospitals do not specifically ask for fresh RBCs, it might be advisable to adopt a quarantine period of 7 days for RBCs (ie, the chosen culture time), to prevent transfusion of possible contaminated units. On the other hand, due to the storage conditions of RBCs, it is very unlikely that bacteria in 7-day-old RBCs have already proliferated to a harmful level for the recipient.

Follow-up in Clinic

In case of a positive signal from an already transfused Platelet unit (or if one of the related RBC units is already transfused) the attending physician should always be informed. The physician will want to pay special attention to signs of a febrile reaction for some days after the transfusion, due to a possible bacterial infection linked to the transfusion. Also, the blood center should ask the transfusion service for a follow-up report on possible transfusion reactions, to document the frequency of TTBI still occurring after the screening system is in place. In the rare case that a unit of platelets with a rapidly growing bacterium (culture positive within 24 hours) is already transfused to a patient, it is worthwhile to determine the antibiotic-resistance pattern in parallel with the differentiation procedure. Especially if a recipient appears to be infected with gram-negative bacteria or with *S. aureus*, this information can be very important in choosing the best treatment.

Another aspect for follow-up is counseling of donors in cases of contamination with bacteria that may have been introduced because the donor had bacteremia. *Yersinia enterocolitica* is well known in this respect but, in general, for cases with gram-negative bacteria or *S. aureus*, it might be worthwhile to check the donor for persistent bacteremia.

Prolonged Platelet Storage

In the early 1980s, developments in bag technology made it possible to extend the storage of platelets, while maintaining the in-vitro quality at a reasonable level.[32-34] Moreover, several reports showed good in-vivo results. On the basis of these studies, the storage time was extended from 5 to 7 days, in both Europe and the United States. In the meantime, transfusion services and health-care workers started to realize that the frequency of TTBI was relatively high compared to virus transmission. After the extension of the storage time, an increase in the reported number of bacterially contaminated Platelet units prompted the US Food and Drug Administration (FDA) to reduce the storage time for platelets back to 5 days.[35] European countries also returned to the 5-day limit. The risk for TTBI presumably increases with storage time, and most of the severe cases of TTBI are associated with platelets stored for 3 days or more.[7] In the meantime, storage containers for platelets have improved and the in-vitro quality of platelets during prolonged storage has likewise improved.[36] Also, platelets stored in a platelet additive solution (which still contains 30% to 40% plasma) maintain the in-vitro quality of platelets for at least 7 days of storage.[37,38] However, although the main obstacle preventing longer storage is the concern about bacterial safety, clinical efficacy must also be demonstrated. In contrast to the situation in the 1980s, good in-vitro data alone are no longer enough to make a component acceptable for transfusion; the principle of evidence-based transfusion is increasingly applied. Therefore, formal clinical trials are necessary to show that extended platelet storage is possible. On the basis of limited data available from clinical studies, the clinical efficacy of platelets stored for 7 days appears similar to that of platelets stored for 5 days, but less than that of fresh platelets (stored 1 - 2 days).[39,40] Large studies will be necessary to prove that the difference between 5 and 7 days is insignificant. These studies should not only compare corrected count increments at 1 and 24 hours following platelet transfusion, but also monitor transfusion intervals and the number of Platelet units transfused.

The reported cases of severe or fatal TTBI are mostly caused by bacteria that are easily detected in the first 3 days of culturing and, therefore, could be prevented by a screening system in place.[1,5,9] Screening can be combined with a quarantine period, but this is not necessary. It is unlikely that bacteria will grow faster in the Platelet unit stored at 22 C than in the sample aliquot in the optimal culture medium at 35 to 37 C. For this reason, a "negative to date" release system works very well.

Upon prolongation of storage time to 7 days or even longer, one should be aware of transmission of slow-growing bacteria, such as *Propionibacterium* species. So far, these bacteria are not seen as very harmful to the recipient and few cases have been reported with fatal outcomes after transmission of *Propionibacterium* species.[1,5] However, this type of contamination might become a problem during extended storage because the units would no longer be transfused before reaching the threshold for inducing TTBI in the recipient.

Cost-Effectiveness

With respect to cost-effectiveness of introducing a system of bacterial screening for blood products, there are two aspects: 1) the amount saved by preventing TTBI vs costs of screening, and 2) the amount saved by prolonged storage vs costs of screening. The first aspect can be calculated only by using several estimates. The second aspect can be considered as a possible savings only because extension of shelf-life to 7 days is not yet generally allowed.

The costs for bacterial screening of platelets in The Netherlands are about EUR19 (US$22) per Platelet unit, including all costs for confirmation, recall procedures, wastage of associated RBC units, etc. Because of the short shelf life for platelets, the outdating is very high and estimated at 25% (based on figures for The Netherlands). Thus, the cost per transfused unit is higher.

On the basis of data in the literature, a rough estimate is that about one of six bacterially contaminated units transfused will result in TTBI.[1,10] The mortality rate associated with these cases is about 15%.[8] Translated from a true-positive rate of about 1 per 2000 per Platelet unit,[6] this will result in about eight cases of severe TTBI per 100,000 transfused apheresis platelets and about 40 cases per 100,000 for pools of whole-blood-derived platelets. The number of fatalities per year per 100,000 transfused units will be one to two for apheresis platelets and about six for platelets from whole blood donations. Although it is very easy to calculate much lower or higher numbers using different literature data, the clinical data based on large numbers of transfusions[9] are very close to the calculated numbers above. With the assumption that bacterial screening will prevent TTBI for >95% of contaminated units and the assumption that costs of treatment for a severe TTBI in the order of EUR10,000 (US$11,700), the costs for preventing one death by screening will be about EUR300,000 (US$351,000) in case of pooled platelet components. In these calculations, no value is given to the improved quality of life for patients prevented from getting TTBI with all the consequences. Instead of costs per prevented death, it is also possible to calculate the costs per prevented TTBI; this will be around EUR57,000 (US$66,900) for whole-blood-derived platelets and around EUR280,000 (US$327,600) for apheresis platelets.

From the screening results in The Netherlands, it can be estimated that the true-positive rate for relevant bacteria (mainly the ones resulting in a positive culture within 3 days, thus excluding *Propionibacterium* and *Corynebacterium* species) is about 1 per 1000 apheresis units. Using the same approach as above, the cost per prevented TTBI case or TTBI-associated death will be lower, but because accurate clinical data on the number of TTBI cases before introduction of the screening are not available, this will never be proven.

The calculation with respect to cost-effectiveness of bacterial screening if used as an instrument to allow extension of shelf life is much easier. By extending the shelf life, the outdating can be reduced substantially, resulting in 1) saving the costs of thousands of Platelet units [production costs EUR130 (US$152) per pooled unit] that would no longer be discarded, and 2) saving costs of screening these units. In practice, it was found that outdating can be reduced from 25% to 10% (Hinloopen B, personal communication). With this reduction, the saving of production costs is already equal to the total costs for the screening system before the extension of shelf life, whereas upon extension of shelf life, the costs of screening per transfused Platelet unit will be reduced about 25%. Because the production costs of apheresis platelets are higher than those of whole-blood-derived platelets, the break-even point in the case of extended shelf life for apheresis platelets can be reached at a lower reduction in outdating rate. In the United States, with about two-thirds of platelet transfusions given as apheresis platelets, 18% of units are reported as outdated; in contrast, when 7-day storage was allowed, this rate was as low as 5%.[39]

Therefore, implementation of bacterial screening in combination with extension of storage time will allow improvement of patient safety with minimal—if any—additional costs. This is in sharp contrast with such measures as the introduction of NAT for HIV and HCV. For additional measures to reduce the risk of TTBI (improved donor arm cleansing and/or diversion of first donor volume), the cost-effectiveness will be lower. Improved donor arm cleansing and/or diversion of the initial collection will principally reduce gram-positive organisms. However, the use of a detection system will protect the recipient against both gram-positive and gram-negative organisms. This is particularly important, given that gram-negative organisms are found in only a small fraction of the contaminated units, but are responsible for the majority of the fatalities related to bacterial contamination.[8,9]

References

1. Sazama K. Reports on 355 transfusion-associated deaths: 1976 through 1985. Transfusion 1990;30:583-90.

2. Blajchman MA, Ali AM. Bacteria in the blood supply: An overlooked issue in transfusion medicine. In: Blood safety: Current challenges. Bethesda, MD: American Association of Blood Banks, 1992:213-28.
3. de Korte D, Marcelis JH, Soeterboek AM. Determination of the degree of bacterial contamination of whole-blood collections using an automated microbe-detection system. Transfusion 2001;41:815-18.
4. Busch MP, Kleinman SH, Nemo GJ. Current and emerging infectious risks of blood transfusion. JAMA 2003;289:959-62.
5. Wagner SJ, Friedman LI, Dodd RY. Transfusion-associated bacterial sepsis. Clin Microbiol Rev 1994;7:290-302.
6. Blajchman MA, Ali AM, Lyn P. Bacterial surveillance of platelet concentrates: Quantitation of bacterial load (abstract). Transfusion 1997; 37(Suppl):74S.
7. Morrow JF, Braine HG. Septic reactions to platelet transfusion, a persistent problem. JAMA 1991;266:555-8.
8. Perez P, Salmi LR, Folléa G, et al. Determinants of transfusion-associated bacterial contamination: Results of the French BACTHEM case-control study. Transfusion 2001;41:862-72.
9. Ness PM, Braine HG, King K, et al. Single-donor platelets reduce the risk of septic platelet transfusion reactions. Transfusion 2001;41:857-61.
10. Yomtovian R. Novel methods for detection of platelet bacterial contamination. Vox Sang 2002;83(Suppl 1):129-31.
11. Goldman M, Roy G, Fréchette N, et al. Evaluation of donor skin disinfection methods. Transfusion 1997;37:309-12.
12. Lee CK, Hin PL, Mak A, et al. Impact of donor arm skin disinfection on the bacterial contamination rate of platelet concentrates. Vox Sang 2002;83:204-8.
13. McDonald CP, Lowe P, Roy A, et al. Evaluation of donor arm disinfection techniques. Vox Sang 2001;80:135-41.
14. Bruneau C, Perez P, Chassaigne M, et al. Efficacy of a new collection procedure for preventing bacterial contamination of whole-blood donations. Transfusion 2001;41:74-81.
15. Wagner SJ, Robinette D, Friedman LI, et al. Diversion of initial blood flow to prevent whole-blood contamination by skin surface bacteria: An in vitro model. Transfusion 2000;40:335-8.
16. de Korte D, Marcelis JH, Verhoeven AJ, et al. Diversion of first blood volume results in a reduction of bacterial contamination for whole-blood collections. Vox Sang 2002;83:13-16.
17. Liu H-W, Cheng TSY, Lee KB, et al. Reduction of platelet transfusion-associated sepsis by short-term bacterial culture. Vox Sang 1999;77:1-5.
18. Björk P, Johnson U. Detection of bacterial growth in platelet concentrates (abstract). Vox Sang 1998;74(Suppl):1267.
19. Schelstraete B, Bijnens BJ, Wuyts G. Prevalence of bacteria in leukodepleted pooled platelet concentrates and apheresis platelets: A 3-year experience (abstract). Transfusion 2000;40(Suppl):12S.

20. Goldman M, Sher G, Blajchman MA. Bacterial contamination of cellular blood products: The Canadian perspective. Transfus Sci 2000; 23:17-19.
21. Sen K, Asher DM. Multiplex PCR for detection of *Enterobacteriaceae* in blood. Transfusion 2001;41:1356-64.
22. Brecher ME, Wong ECC, Chen SE, et al. Antibiotic-labeled probes and microvolume fluorimetry for the rapid detection of bacterial contamination in platelet components: A preliminary report. Transfusion 2000; 40:411-13.
23. Brecher ME, Hogan JJ, Boothe G, et al. Platelet bacterial contamination and the use of a chemiluminescence-linked universal bacterial ribosomal RNA gene probe. Transfusion 1994;34:750-5.
24. Seaver M, Crookston JC, Roselle DC, et al. First results using automated epifluorescence microscopy to detect *Escherichia coli* and *Staphylococcus epidermidis* in WBC-reduced platelet concentrates. Transfusion 2001;41:1351-5.
25. Thorpe TC, Wilson ML, Turner JE, et al. BacT/ALERT: An automated microbial detection system. J Clin Microbiol 1990;28:1608-12.
26. McDonald CP, Smith R, Calvin J, et al. Evaluation of the Pall bacterial detection system (BDS) (abstract). Vox Sang 2002;83(Suppl 2):7.
27. Castro E, Bueno JL. Bacterial contamination of blood components needs to be confirmed. Transfusion 2002;42:380-1.
28. Brecher ME, Means N, Jere CS, et al. Evaluation of an automated culture system for detecting bacterial contamination of platelets: An analysis with 15 contaminating organisms. Transfusion 2001;41:477-82.
29. Brecher ME, Heath DG, Hay SN, et al. Evaluation of a new generation of culture bottle using an automated bacterial culture system for detecting nine common contaminating organisms found in platelet components. Transfusion 2002;42:774-9.
30. Laport R, Bakker M, van Schayk A, et al. Detection of bacterial contamination of platelet concentrates. Presented at VI Regional ISBT meeting, Tel Aviv, Israel, May 8-12, 1999.
31. Van Haute I, Van Vooren M, Lootens N, et al. Screening of platelet concentrates for bacterial growth (abstract). Transfusion 2000;40(Suppl): 70S.
32. Hogge DE, Thompson BW, Schiffer CA. Platelet storage for 7 days in second-generation blood bags. Transfusion 1986;26:131-5.
33. Holme S, Heaton WA, Courtright M. Improved in vivo and in vitro viability of platelet concentrates stored for seven days in a platelet additive solution. Br J Haematol 1987;66:233-8.
34. Simon TL, Nelson EJ, Murphy S. Extension of platelet concentrate storage to 7 days in second-generation bags. Transfusion 1987;27:6-9.
35. Food and Drug Administration. Memorandum: Reduction of the maximal platelet storage period to 5 days in an approved container (February, 1986).
36. Kostelijk EH, Gouwerok CWN, Veldman H, et al. Comparison between a new PVC platelet storage container (UPX80) and a polyolefin container. Transfus Med 2000;10:131-9.

37. Gulliksson H, Sallander S, Pedajas I, et al. Storage of platelets in additive solutions: A new method for storage using sodium chloride solution. Transfusion 1992;32:435-40.
38. Heaton WA, Holme S, Keegan T. Development of a combined storage medium for 7-day storage of platelet concentrates and 42-day storage of red cell concentrates. Br J Haematol 1990;75:400-7.
39. AuBuchon JP, Cooper LK, Leach MF, et al. Experience with universal bacterial culturing to detect contamination of apheresis platelet units in a hospital transfusion service. Transfusion 2002;42:855-61.
40. Dijkstra-Tiekstra MJ, Hendriks ECM, van der Meer P, et al. Clinical effectiveness of leukodepleted platelet concentrates that were stored for up to 7 days (abstract). Vox Sang 2002;83(Suppl 2):7.

In: Brecher ME, ed.
Bacterial and Parasitic Contamination of Blood Components
Bethesda, MD: AABB Press, 2003

5

Transfusion-Transmitted Syphilis

RITCHARD G. CABLE, MD, AND
SHARYN ORTON, PHD

THE ASSOCIATION BETWEEN SYPHILIS AND the spirochete *Treponema pallidum* was first described in 1905 with the demonstration of spirochetes in Giemsa-stained fluid from a syphilitic lesion.[1] Person-to-person transmission primarily occurs during sexual intercourse but may also be transmitted congenitally or by blood

Ritchard G. Cable, MD, Medical Director, American Red Cross, Connecticut Blood Services, Farmington, Connecticut, and Sharyn Orton, PhD, Special Assistant to the Director, Division of Blood Applications, Office of Blood Research and Review, Center for Biologics Evaluation and Research, Food and Drug Administration, Rockville, Maryland

(The views of the authors represent scientific opinions and should not be construed as opinion or policy of the United States Food and Drug Administration or other institutions with which the authors are affiliated.)

transfusion.[2] Studies indicated that transfusion-associated syphilis occurred in almost every case when fresh infectious blood was transfused.[3]

Early in the 20th century, syphilis was a major public health problem, with the first case of transfusion-transmitted syphilis described in 1915. In 1938, a serologic test for syphilis (STS) was initiated as the first infectious disease test performed on blood donations. By 1941, 138 cases of transfusion-transmitted syphilis had been described in the literature.[4] Today, transfusion-transmitted syphilis has become nonexistent in the United States, with the last case being reported in 1969.[5] This is even more remarkable, given that 1) there was increased demand for fresh, although refrigerated, blood in the early 1990s,[3] 2) the syphilis spirochete can be found in the blood during the seronegative phase,[5] 3) the transfusion of blood components occurs early in storage associated with low blood inventories, and 4) the use of platelet concentrates has increased.

Epidemiology of Syphilis in the United States

In 1947 before the discovery and use of penicillin, the incidence of primary and secondary syphilis was 66.4 cases per 100,000 persons.[1] The discovery of penicillin therapy and extensive public health efforts in the 1940s decreased the incidence rate of syphilis to only 3.9 cases per 100,000 population in 1956. The last syphilis epidemic occurred in 1990, when the incidence was 20.3 per 100,000 persons. This was the highest rate in the United States since the 1940s, and disproportionately affected Blacks, who had rates 60-fold higher than Whites. Age, marital status, urban residence, race, ethnicity, socioeconomic status, and sexual or drug behavior were also factors in this epidemic. By 1993, the rate had dropped to 10.4 per 100,000.[6]

The incidence rate of syphilis continued a steady decline between 1995 (6.3 cases per 100,000 population[7]) and 2000 (2.1 cases per 100,000 population[8]). However, in 2001, the syphilis rate increased slightly to 2.2 cases per 100,000 population (0.7

in non-Hispanic Whites; 12.2 in non-Hispanic Blacks; 1.6 in Hispanics).[8] Compared to the year 2000, 2001 rates increased in non-Hispanic Whites by 40%; Hispanics by 31%; Asian/Pacific Islanders by 67%; American Indian/Alaska Natives by 75%; and men (15% overall). Rates declined in non-Hispanic Blacks by 10% and women (18% overall). The highest rate was in the South (56% of all cases), although this was a decrease from the previous year. Rates also decreased 10% in the Midwest but increased 40% in the West and 57% in the Northeast. In 2001, no cases were reported in 80% of United States counties and an additional 0.5% of counties reported rates less than or equal to 0.2 cases per 100,000 population. Twenty counties and one city accounted for 51% of all reported cases. The counties/cities with the highest case rates were Robeson County, North Carolina; Fulton County, Georgia (Atlanta); Baltimore, Maryland; and Shelby County, Tennessee (Memphis). Rates were still disproportionally higher in non-Hispanic Blacks compared with non-Hispanic Whites.[8]

During the past decade, the crack cocaine epidemic and associated increase in sex exchanged for drugs,[9] and male sex with another male (MSM)[10] have become the primary factors contributing to the syphilis epidemic. From the data collected for 2001, the increase was attributable exclusively to outbreaks in MSM. These outbreaks were also associated with high rates of co-infection with the human immunodeficiency virus (HIV) and high-risk sexual behavior among specific subgroups of MSM.[8]

Clinical and Diagnostic Considerations

Syphilis usually is acquired following sexual contact with an infected individual. Typically, the first sign of syphilis is a chancre, a small painless indurated ulcer, which usually occurs on the genitals but can occur also in the mouth and anal mucosa. Rarely, the lesion appears in other areas where contact of abraded skin with another person's chancre can inoculate the *T. pallidum* spirochete. The chancre usually appears 3 to 90 days (average 21 days) after contact.[11] *T. pallidum* disseminates from the primary chancre through the blood, although the timing of spirochetemia in primary syphilis and its relationship to the serologic "window" is not well characterized. However, spirochetemia can occur early because transmission by transfusion has been reported in this serologic "window."[11]

Secondary syphilis is usually manifested as a disseminated erythematous rash appearing approximately 2 to 8 weeks after the chancre.[11] Spirochetemia appears to be most intense during secondary syphilis, and the rash is believed to be caused by local deposition in the skin of the spirochete along with the associated immune reaction. If untreated, the rash of secondary syphilis fades and the disease enters a latent phase, where the patient becomes seropositive but asymptomatic. The latent period may last from a few months to many years. Relapse, particularly mucocutaneous relapse, can occur within 4 years after initial infection, implying that the patient is infectious during the early years of latency.[11] Later manifestations of residual disease are called late or tertiary syphilis, characterized by local tissue damage with associated symptoms. Although almost any organ can be involved with tertiary syphilis, the disease classically affects the heart and the nervous system (neurosyphilis), often with significant morbidity or death. Tertiary syphilis can produce manifestations decades after the initial infection. It is difficult to eradicate the spirochete in tertiary syphilis. Spirochetemia is believed to occur in tertiary syphilis, although the evidence for this phenomenon is less well documented than during secondary syphilis or during early relapse.[11]

It is assumed that transfusion-transmitted syphilis occurs from the transmission of spirochetes from the blood of the blood donor to that of the recipient. Characterizing the spirochetemia in a patient with syphilis has been greatly complicated by the inability to grow *T. pallidum* in culture. *T. pallidum* is an extremely fastidious organism and, except for an experimental tissue culture system,[12] usually is identified by dark field examination of swabs from clinical lesions. Syphilis cannot be cultured under standard laboratory conditions, although it can be grown by injecting infectious material into a rabbit's testicle or intradermally, resulting in a typical dark field positive lesion containing *T. pallidum.*[11]

Except for dark field examination of clinical chancres for spirochetes, the primary basis for the diagnosis of syphilis is serologic. A short summary of the available methods[13-15] follows.

Two separate approaches to serologic diagnosis exist. In the first approach, the development of high titers of antibodies to cardiolipin and other phospholipids in patients with active syphilis is the basis for a large variety of serologic methods. The classic method is the Venereal Disease Research Laboratory (VDRL) test, and the most commonly used method is the rapid plasma reagin (RPR) test. The latter test is available as a manual card test and in several automated formats. These methods use a complex lipid antigen called cardiolipin to detect the nonspecific "reaginic" antibodies that develop in high titer in patients with active syphilis. The cardiolipin-based tests are easy to perform and have the additional advantage of reflecting clinical disease activity in the antibody titer.

Unfortunately, the cardiolipin tests are nonspecific and are often positive in patients with autoimmune or other infectious diseases (biologic false positive). More recently, as a second approach to STS, an automated screening test has been implemented in the United States for blood donor screening that is based on detection of specific antibody to treponemal antigens with a hemagglutination endpoint (PK-TP, Olympus Corporation, Lake Success, NY). However, there is a significant prevalence of false-positive tests in normal healthy blood donors with both screening tests. Consequently, it is standard practice to perform specific treponemal antibody testing on all blood donors who have a positive STS of either test type. The usual confirmatory test is the fluorescent treponemal antigen-absorbed (FTA-ABS) test,[11] although several other methods exist.[15] It should be noted that because the FTA-ABS and PK-TP tests both use treponemal antigens, they are not together an ideal "confirmation system." Many laboratories test PK-TP-positive donors with the RPR test, as well as with the FTA-ABS test. However, because the RPR test disappears more quickly after treatment, a result that is PK-TP positive, FTA-ABS positive, and RPR negative is not considered a false-positive result, but rather a serologic residue of a previous syphilis infection.

Transfusion-Transmitted Syphilis

Because *T. pallidum* is a fragile organism, it does not tolerate prolonged storage. The most thorough studies of survival of *T. pallidum* in stored blood were conducted by Van der Sluis et al,[16,17] who concluded that the spirochete can survive for up to 5 days under refrigerated blood bank storage conditions. The effect of storage on *T. pallidum* is further discussed below.

With control of syphilis by modern public health and treatment approaches, reported transfusion-transmitted syphilis has all but disappeared.[18] Only two cases of transfusion-transmitted syphilis have been reported in the English literature since 1965. Chambers et al[5] described a 28-year-old male with lymphoma who developed secondary syphilis following the transfusion of six Red Blood Cell (RBC) units and 25 "fresh" platelet concentrates that were screened with the VDRL test. Twenty-two of 25 platelet donors could be retested and all were STS negative. The authors attributed the syphilis to one of the three untested platelet donors. Risseeuw-Appel and Kothe[19] described syphilis in a full-term newborn after exchange transfusion with "fresh" whole blood. The donor was STS negative 5 days before donation and STS positive 5 months after donation.

When a disease is reported as rarely as transfusion-transmitted syphilis, clinicians are unlikely to recognize a case when it occurs. In fact, transfusion-transmitted syphilis may be more common than reported. Because it is difficult to exclude sexually transmitted syphilis, transfusion cases may be excluded erroneously. Transfusion cases have no chancre, which is the diagnostic hallmark of syphilis. Moreover, many transfusion recipients are treated with antibiotics coincidentally. This may prevent syphilis or modify the clinical picture so that it is unrecognizable.

The Effects of Blood Component Production and Storage on the Viability of Syphilis

Several hypotheses have been put forward to explain the lack of reports of transfusion-transmitted syphilis, including the impact of refrigeration on the survival of the spirochete.[20] Preparation and storage of individual blood components may have an impact on the potential for transfusion transmission.

Experimental inoculation of whole blood, coupled with rabbit inoculation tests of the stored inoculated blood, has shown that the infectious potential of whole blood stored at 4 C is directly proportional to the size of the inoculum. Inoculum concentrations of 5.0×10^4 treponemes/mL, 1.25×10^6 treponemes/mL, and 2.5×10^7 treponemes/mL were able to induce syphilis in rabbits detectable up to 36 hours, 72 hours, and 108 hours after storage at 4 C, respectively.[16,17] However, these inoculation concentrations were assumed by the authors to be unrealistically high relative to the number of organisms expected to be present in the peripheral circulation of infected individuals,[17] and the studies were limited to 4 C storage of whole blood. In fact, the concentration of treponemes in the blood of a naturally infected individual at different phases of infection (from preliminary data on five blood samples from individuals studied in a syphilis outbreak in Maricopa County, Arizona) suggests that the concentration varies from approximately 50 to 100,000 organisms/mL, depending on the phase of infection.[21]

In experiments designed to characterize the compartmentalization of the spirochete into blood components, three units of whole blood were experimentally inoculated with 10^4, 10^5, and 10^6 organisms/mL and processed into RBCs, platelet concentrates, and Fresh Frozen Plasma (FFP).[22] The RBCs were split into two aliquots, one stored at 4 C and one at 25 C (room temperature) for 24 hours. Samples were tested for *T. pallidum* RNA[23] and DNA[24] and the concentration of organism per component determined.[24] *T. pallidum* DNA and RNA could be detected in all components, with 64% to 84% of the inoculated organism detected in the RBCs, 3% to 21% in the FFP, and 13% to 19% in the platelets. The concentration of treponemes per milliliter was highest in the platelet concentrates and lowest in the FFP.[22]

This work was further expanded to include rabbit inoculation testing to assess the potential for infectivity. Whole blood units were inoculated with 10^1 to 10^5 organisms/mL and split into two aliquots for storage at 4 C and 25 C. Samples were taken over 3 days, and infectivity was determined by intradermal inoculation into the backs of rabbits. Diminished infectivity was observed at 4 C compared with 25 C relative to time and concentration.[25] It is unknown if this decrease in infectivity is directly related to the effect of temperature or whether other variables not yet determined (ie, the presence or absence of viable white cells) have an impact. Regardless, because current transfusion demands for red cells often lead to the transfusion of blood that is only a few days old, it cannot be assumed that storage at 4 C would preclude transfusion transmission of this agent.[20]

Evidence that the *T. pallidum* spirochete attaches to the surface membrane of phagocytes[26] may have implications in view of the increased use of leukocyte reduction filters. The transfusion medicine field is debating the medical value of a policy of universal leukocyte reduction of all cellular blood components (ie, RBCs and platelets) for the removal of white cells. Universal leukocyte reduction may decrease the potential for transfusion-transmitted syphilis.

Platelets are stored in bags designed to facilitate oxygen transport. This property of currently used platelet containers leads to an internal oxygen content (10 - 15%)[27,28] that is higher than the *T. pallidum* spirochete can withstand (1 - 4%[29]). Thus, the level of oxygen tension in platelet containers in use today is likely to cause the death of the organism,[3] although the actual impact on survival time is unknown.

Should We Test for Syphilis in Blood Donors?—A Regulatory History

Although blood banks have tested for syphilis in blood donors since the early days of blood banking, in 1985, the requirement for syphilis testing was removed from the American Association of Blood Banks (AABB) *Standards for Blood Banks and Transfusion Services*. This change was not supported by the Food and Drug Administration (FDA). The FDA's position at that time was that STS be retained as a potential surrogate for high-risk behavior for HIV infection rather than as evidence of syphilis, and syphilis screening continued to be a mandatory requirement. In 1995, the National Institutes of Health (NIH) convened a Consensus Development Conference,[20] which included discussion of the extent to which tests for syphilis contributed to transfusion safety, and whether their use as in current practice should be continued or modified. The resulting recommendations were to continue syphilis screening of all blood donors until such time as 1) more information was obtained regarding the effect of component storage conditions on *T. pallidum* survival, and 2) molecular techniques could be used to assess the absence of *T. pallidum* in serologically positive donated blood.[20]

The value of syphilis testing in blood donors was most recently revisited after the FDA released proposed rules in 1999.[30] The FDA specifically requested data addressing the value of donor testing for syphilis 1) as a marker of high-risk behavior, 2) as a surrogate test for other infectious diseases, and 3) in preventing the transmission of syphilis through blood transfusion. At that time, public health officials also noted that syphilis screening of blood donors had resulted in the identification of a small number of previously unreported cases of syphilis.[31] The pros and cons of testing blood donors for syphilis are summarized in Table 5-1.

Table 5-1. Some Pros and Cons of Donor Screening for Syphilis

Pros

- The rarity of posttransfusion syphilis may be due, in part, to screening.
- There may be public health value in identifying a small number of cases of previously unrecognized syphilis.
- Testing avoids passive transmission of a high-titer donor treponemal antibody, which could cause a positive STS without infection in the recipient, confusing clinical management.
- There may be value for the STS as a surrogate test for newly emergent sexually and transfusion-transmitted diseases.
- Testing is required by the Food and Drug Administration.

Cons

- Syphilis testing costs money.
- Nonspecificity of tests results in a significant discard rate.
- Known causes of a false-positive STS appear not to apply to a blood donor population. The significance of a false-positive syphilis screening test result in a donor is unknown.
- Donors with false-positive STS are often alarmed and inconvenienced.
- Seropositive donors with adequate treatment for previous syphilis are often embarrassed and inappropriately deferred.
- Syphilis is rarely transmitted by blood transfusion.
- Current testing is not perfect—window period cases may occur.

Since the 1995 Consensus Development Conference and the 1999 proposed FDA rules, additional information has been acquired to address the questions posed by the FDA. That information is summarized below. Recently, the proposed FDA regulations have been made final and continue to require the testing of blood donors for syphilis.[32]

Recent Data on the Limited Surrogate Value of a Positive Syphilis Test

The value of the STS as a surrogate test for HIV, hepatitis B virus (HBV), and hepatitis C virus (HCV) is suggested by seroprevalence studies in which testing for all four markers is performed on populations at high risk for disease. A significant correlation between the STS and HIV has been found in patients treated at sexually transmitted disease (STD) clinics.[33] Significant correlation between HIV and syphilis serology has also been seen in intravenous drug users[34] and homosexual men.[35] Primary or secondary syphilis was highly correlated with subsequent seroconversion to HIV in a population in a Florida STD clinic,[36] suggesting the possibility that syphilitic lesions facilitate the transmission of HIV.[35] A correlation between seropositivity for syphilis and HBV in prostitutes is equally well established,[37] and a similar correlation for HCV has been suggested for STD clinic patients.[38]

The "window period donor" is believed to represent a significant threat to the safety of the blood supply. Definitive proof of the value of syphilis serology as a surrogate test for HIV and other transfusion-transmitted viruses would require a large study of the STS in donors seroconverting for these markers. Although this has not been done, Herrara et al[39] evaluated HIV- and STS-positive blood donations in 16 Red Cross blood centers among 4,500,000 blood donations during 1992-1994. Of the total, 12,145 donations (0.27%) were STS positive and 377 (0.008%) were HIV positive. Among donations that were negative on the other screening tests, STS-positive donations were 12 times more likely to be HIV positive (odds ratio 11.9; 95% CI 5-26). However, of an estimated 13 HIV infectious window period donations during this period, only 0.2 would have been removed solely by a positive STS. Similar results were found for the surrogate potential of the STS to prevent the other transfusion-transmitted viruses.[39] With the addition of HIV and HCV nucleic acid amplification testing (NAT) in routine blood bank testing, the number of residual HCV and

HIV infectious donations interdicted by STS testing is even smaller.

Thus, despite the strong association between the seroprevalence of syphilis and the seroprevalence of HIV, HBV, and HCV, it appears that syphilis testing has very limited utility as a surrogate test for these viruses in a volunteer donor population in the United States. This is because of diminishing returns. The prevalence of these diseases has already been greatly reduced by improvements in donor screening and serologic and NAT testing. It is possible, however, that experience in other countries may be different because of the higher viral infection rate in these donor populations and the limited availability of screening tests. It is also possible that the STS may have future value as a surrogate test in the United States blood donor population if another undiscovered transfusion-associated and sexually transmitted pathogen appears in the blood supply.

Recent Data on the Presence of *T. pallidum* in Serologically Positive Blood Components

A recent case series[23] described *T. pallidum* DNA and RNA testing of 169 STS-reactive, FTA-ABS-confirmed-positive aliquots from the platelet concentrates of volunteer blood donors. The series included 48 RPR positive donors (compatible with recent or active disease). No sample contained *T. pallidum* DNA or RNA.[23] This pilot study suggests that there is a low (0 - 3%) probability that the blood of donors who have confirmed positive syphilis test results is infectious for syphilis. Unfortunately, the confidence interval from such a small pilot study is rather wide. A definitive assessment of the incidence of *T. pallidum* transfusion transmission in the current transfusion environment will likely require a larger study. Such a study, with no infected blood components identified, may provide useful data in favor of eliminating the requirement for testing. Because other factors continue to influence the decision to retain the requirement for syphilis testing, it is unlikely the costs of a study of the required size will be undertaken. Thus, the question of whether syphilis is transmissible under today's blood banking conditions remains unanswered.

Recent Data on the Benefit of Syphilis Screening of Blood Donors on Community Case Finding and the Control of Syphilis in the United States

Blood banks are required, as are other laboratories that screen for syphilis, to report confirmed positive test results to state and/or local health departments for the purpose of contacting the donor, ensuring they receive adequate treatment, and tracing sexual contacts of the positive donor, so that they, too, can be tested and evaluated for treatment. Gardella et al[40] recently published the Centers for Disease Control and Prevention (CDC) findings, showing that during 1995 to 2000 inclusive, 22 primary, 81 secondary, and 413 early latent syphilis cases were identified through blood/plasma donor screening in 16 states. Of these donors, 58% were volunteer donors and 42% paid plasma donors. After adjustment for reporting system differences, the authors project that approximately 200 cases of early syphilis per year were detected in the United States by blood bank screening. Approximately 100 of these would be volunteer donors, who the authors conclude may be at risk for transmitting syphilis. The authors also state that syphilis screening of blood donors may have "broader, albeit secondary public health implications." The authors reference the CDC's *National Plan to Eliminate Syphilis from the United States*.[41] Although the plan does not specifically call for blood bank screening for syphilis, the authors suggest that blood donor screening and subsequent follow-up may augment efforts to eliminate syphilis. Syphilis cases identified through blood/plasma donor screening, however, only accounted for 0.4% of all primary/secondary and 1.0% of early latent cases reported during the 6-year study.

STS and Blood Donation—Implications for the Donor

Approximately 25,000 donors per year in the United States have reactive STS results, and only 40% confirm positive by FTA-ABS.[23] It is unclear if the testing algorithms used by blood banks are truly identifying any currently infected donors. To what can we attribute confirmed and unconfirmed positive (false-positive) syphilis test results in blood donors? Many confirmed positive syphilis tests in donors are a result of past, treated syphilis infection. This may be particularly true of donors identified with a primary treponemal-based antigen test.

There are also many clinical conditions associated with false-positive syphilis test results, using both cardiolipin-based and treponemal-based test systems in a clinical environment.[11,42-44] To determine if these clinical conditions applied in the setting of blood donor screening with the PK-TP test system, a case control study of donors with reactive (both FTA-ABS confirmed and nonconfirmed) and nonreactive PK-TP test results was conducted. Data were collected via an anonymous mail survey regarding a history of conditions reported to be associated with FP syphilis tests and/or a previous history of syphilis infection.[45] Among survey respondents, approximately 50% of donors with FTA-ABS-positive test results reported a syphilis history. There was no statistically significant difference in the frequency of other reported clinical conditions, associated in the literature with false-positive STS test results, for donors with either FTA-ABS-positive (confirmed) or FTA-ABS-negative (unconfirmed) test results, compared with controls.[45]

These results demonstrate that: 1) Approximately half of confirmed PK-TP-positive test results are a result of past, treated, syphilis infection; 2) Conditions historically reported in the literature as being associated with false-positive test results do not appear to explain false-positive PK-TP test results in healthy blood donors; and 3) Although no donor with a PK-TP-positive, FTA-ABS-negative test status reported a history of syphilis, it is unclear if the half of donors who had a PK-TP-positive, FTA-ABS-positive test result, but did not report a history of syphilis, were currently infected or had a previous history of syphilis infection, known or unknown to them.[45]

Designing counseling strategies or informational material for blood donors with a positive STS test is extremely difficult, given the lack of information about the donor's risk status and sexual history. Donors with confirmed tests for syphilis should be counseled with sensitivity to the possibility that either they have had treated syphilis in the past or they may be unaware of their test status, which may represent current or past syphilis. Donors with false-positive test results can be counseled as not being infected with syphilis.

In both situations, the advice to the donor regarding subsequent blood donation is problematic. Confirmed STS-positive donors are eligible to donate again 12 months after a confirmed positive donation, with completion of necessary syphilis treatment, as long as evidence of evaluation by the donor's physician is provided. The rationale for the 12-month deferral is primarily to serve as a surrogate for high-risk behavior.[46] Many of these donors will continue to be confirmed STS positive on subsequent donations. The donor with a false-positive STS can be encouraged to donate again, but many blood centers defer such donors temporarily, or permanently if the false-positive STS test is persistent, to reduce the possibility of another false-positive donation.

Future Developments

National Plan to Eliminate Syphilis in the United States

One way to reduce the risk of transfusion-transmitted syphilis to near zero, and thus the need for STS screening of blood donors, is the elimination of syphilis in the United States. In October 1999, the CDC National Center for HIV, STD, and TB

Prevention published *The National Plan to Eliminate Syphilis from the United States.*[41] National elimination of syphilis is defined as "the absence of sustained transmission in the United States." Local elimination is defined as "the absence of transmission of new cases within the jurisdiction except within 90 days of report of an imported index case."[41] The overall national goals are to reduce cases of primary and secondary syphilis to 1000 or fewer cases (approximately 0.4 case per 100,000 population) and to increase to 90% the number of counties reporting no cases of syphilis. Geographic focus will primarily target current high morbidity areas and areas with potential for re-emergence of syphilis, with low morbidity areas retaining strong STD prevention programs. The CDC has committed to enhanced surveillance and health promotion, strong community involvement and partnerships, expanded clinical and laboratory services, and rapid outbreak response to ensure the success of this program.[41] Clearly, the lower the prevalence of syphilis in the general population, the lower the prevalence in the donor population, which results in a lower risk of transfusion transmission of syphilis.

Molecular Methods for Syphilis Testing and Risk Assessment

In the absence of test elimination and with the improvement in characterization of *T. pallidum* antigens[47] and complete genomic sequencing,[48] development of an inexpensive, sensitive, specific, automated, test methodology (ie, polymerase chain reaction) for the presence of *T. pallidum* spirochetes would be beneficial because detection of potentially infectious blood components is the primary concern. The development of facile molecular diagnostic methods also may expedite the assessment of the risk of syphilis when collected from a donor who is seropositive for syphilis. Such data, if of sufficient power, may enable the elimination of testing blood donors for syphilis before the eradication of syphilis in the United States.

References

1. Singh AE, Romanowski B. Syphilis: Review with emphasis on clinical, epidemiologic, and some biologic features. Clin Microbiol Rev 1999; 12:187-209.
2. Felman YM, Nikitas JA. Sexually transmitted diseases. Primary syphilis. Cutis 1982;29:122-4,128,133,136.
3. Seidl S. Syphilis screening in the 1990s. Transfusion 1990;30:773-4.
4. Goens JL, Janniger CK, De Wolf K. Dermatologic and systemic manifestations of syphilis. Am Fam Physician 1994;50:1013-20.
5. Chambers RW, Foley HT, Schmidt PJ. Transmission of syphilis by fresh blood components. Transfusion 1969;9:32-4.
6. Kilmarx P. The evolving epidemiology of syphilis (editorial). Am J Public Health 1995;85:1053-4.
7. Division of STD Prevention. Sexually transmitted disease surveillance, 1995. U.S. Department of Health and Human Services, Public Health Service. Atlanta, GA: Centers for Disease Control and Prevention, 1996.
8. Primary and secondary syphilis—United States, 2000-2001. MMWR Morb Mortal Wkly Rep 2002;51:971-3.
9. Kilmarx P, Zaidi A, Thomas J, et al. Sociodemographic factors and the variation in syphilis rates among US counties, 1984 through 1993: An ecological analysis. Am J Public Health 1997;87:1937-43.
10. Thomas J, Kulik A, Schoenbach V. Syphilis in the south: Rural rates surpass urban rates in North Carolina. Am J Public Health 1995; 85:1119-22.
11. Tramont EC. *Treponema pallidum* (syphilis). In: Mandell GL, Bennett JE, Dolin R, eds. Principles and practice of infectious diseases. 5th ed. New York: Churchill Livingstone, 2000:2117-33.
12. Jenkin HM, Sandok PL. In vitro cultivation of *Treponema pallidum*. In: Schell RF, Musher DM, eds. Pathogenesis and immunology of treponemal infection. New York: Marcel Dekker, 1983:71-98.
13. Johnson PC, Farnie MA. Testing for syphilis. Dermatol Clin 1994; 12:9-17.
14. Hart G. Syphilis test in diagnostic and therapeutic decision making. Ann Intern Med 1986;104:368-76.
15. Larsen SA. Syphilis. Clin Lab Med 1989;9:545-57.
16. Van der Sluis JJ, Onvlee PC, Kothe FCHA, et al. Transfusion syphilis, survival of *Treponema pallidum* in donor blood I. Report of an orientating study. Vox Sang 1984;47:197-204.
17. Van der Sluis JJ, ten Kate FJW, Vuzevski VD, et al. Transfusion syphilis, survival of *Treponema pallidum* in donor blood II. Dose dependence of experimentally determined survival times. Vox Sang 1985;49:390-9.
18. De Schryver A, Meheus A. Syphilis and blood transfusion: A global perspective. Transfusion 1990;30:844-7.
19. Risseeuw-Appel IM, Kothe FC. Transfusion syphilis: A case report. Sex Transm Dis 1983;10:200-1.

20. Infectious disease testing for blood transfusions. NIH Consens Statement 1995;13:1-27.
21. Liu H, McCaustland K, Holloway B. Evaluating the concentration of *Treponema pallidum* in blood and body fluids using a semi-quantitative PCR method (abstract). Int J STD AIDS 2001;12(Suppl 2):142-3.
22. Orton SL, Liu H, Tomioka K. Distribution of *Treponema pallidum* spirochete in blood components and the effect of storage (abstract).Transfusion 2001;41(Suppl):13S.
23. Orton SL, Liu H, Dodd RY, Williams AE. Prevalence of circulating *T. pallidum* DNA and RNA in blood donors with confirmed positive syphilis tests. Transfusion 2002;42:94-9.
24. Odes B, Liu H, Johnson S, et al. Molecular cloning of a gene *(polA)* coding for an unusual DNA polymerase I from *Treponema pallidum*. J Med Microbiol 2000;49:657-67.
25. Liu H, Chi K, Cox D, et al. Viability of *Treponema pallidum* in stored blood and implications for blood safety. Presented at the International Conference on Emerging Infectious Diseases, Atlanta, GA: March 24-27, 2002.
26. Brause B, Roberts R. Attachment of virulent *Treponema pallidum* to human mononuclear phagocytes. Br J Vener Dis 1978;54:218-24.
27. Grode G, Miripol J, Garber J, et al. Extended storage of platelets in a new plastic container I. Biochemical and morphological changes. Transfusion 1985;25:204-8.
28. Snyder EL, Aster RH, Heaton A, et al. Five-day storage of platelets in a non-diethylhexyl phthalate-plasticized container. Transfusion 1992; 32:736-41.
29. Fitzgerald TJ. Treponema. In: Balows A, Hausler WJ, eds. Manual of clinical microbiology. 5th ed. Washington, DC: American Society for Microbiology, 1991:567-78.
30. Food and Drug Administration. Proposed rule: Requirements for testing human blood donors for evidence of infection due to communicable disease agents. (August 19, 1999) Fed Regist 1999;64:45339-55.
31. FDA Blood Products Advisory Committee Meeting, Gaithersburg, Maryland, September 15, 2000. [Available at http://www.fda.gov/ohrms/dockets/ac/00/transcripts/3649t2.rtf.]
32. Food and Drug Administration. Final rule: Requirements for testing human blood donors for evidence of infection due to communicable disease agents. (June 11, 2001) Fed Regist 2001;66:31146-65.
33. Quinn TC, Cannon RO, Glasser D, et al. The association of syphilis with risk of human immunodeficiency virus infection in patients attending sexually transmitted disease clinics. Arch Intern Med 1990; 150:1297-302.
34. Nelson KE, Vlahov D, Cohn S, et al. Sexually transmitted diseases in a population of intravenous drug users: Association with seropositivity to the human immunodeficiency virus (HIV). J Infect Dis 1991;164: 457-63.

35. Potterat JJ. Does syphilis facilitate sexual acquisition of HIV? (letter) JAMA 1987;258:473.
36. Otten MW Jr, Zaidi AA, Peterman TA, et al. High rate of HIV seroconversion among patients attending urban sexually transmitted disease clinics. AIDS 1994;8:549-53.
37. Rosenblum L, Darrow W, Witte J, et al. Sexual practices in the transmission of hepatitis B virus and prevalence of hepatitis delta virus infection in female prostitutes in the United States. JAMA 1992;267: 2477-81.
38. Thomas DL, Cannon RO, Shapiro CN, et al. Hepatitis C, hepatitis B, and human immunodeficiency virus infections among non-intravenous drug-using patients attending clinics for sexually transmitted diseases. J Infect Dis 1994;169:990-5.
39. Herrara GA, Lackritz EM, Janssen RS, et al. Serologic test for syphilis as a surrogate marker for human immunodeficiency virus infection among United States blood donors. Transfusion 1997;37:836-40.
40. Gardella C, Marfin AA, Kahn RH, et al. Persons with early syphilis identified through blood or plasma donation screening in the United States. J Infect Dis 2000;185:545-9.
41. The National Plan to Eliminate Syphilis from the United States. Division of STD Prevention; National Center for HIV, STD, and TB Prevention. Atlanta, GA: Centers for Disease Control and Prevention, 1999. [Available at http://www.cdc.gov/stopsyphilis/plan.pdf.]
42. Larsen S, Steiner B, Rudolph A. Laboratory diagnosis and interpretation of tests for syphilis. Clin Microbiol Rev 1995;8:1-21.
43. Cruikshank R. Treponema: Borrelia. In: Cruikshank R, ed. Medical microbiology. 12th ed. New York: Churchill Livingstone, 1973:386-92. [Out of print.]
44. Vila P, Hernandez MC, Lopez-Fernandez MF, Batlle J. Prevalence, follow-up and clinical significance of the anticardiolipin antibodies in normal subjects. Thromb Haemost 1994;72:209-313.
45. Orton SL, Dodd RY, Williams AE. Absence of risk factors for false positive test results in blood donors with PK™TP reactive test results for syphilis. Transfusion 2001;41:744-50.
46. Food and Drug Administration Memorandum: Clarification of FDA recommendations for donor deferral and product distribution based on the result of syphilis testing. (December 12, 1992) Rockville, MD: CBER Office of Communication, Training, and Manufacturers Assistance, 1992.
47. Norris S. Polypeptides of *Treponema pallidum*: Progress toward understanding their structural, functional, and immunologic roles. Microbiol Rev 1993;57:750-79.
48. Fraser C, Norris S, Weinstock G, et al. Complete genome sequence of *Treponema pallidum*, the syphilis spirochete. Science 1998;28:375-88.

In: Brecher ME, ed.
Bacterial and Parasitic Contamination of Blood Components
Bethesda, MD: AABB Press, 2003

6

Transfusion-Induced Malaria

LOUIS M. KATZ, MD

MALARIA IS A PROTOZOAN PARASITIC DISEASE caused in humans by four species of the genus *Plasmodium* (*P. falciparum*, *P. vivax*, *P. ovale*, and *P. malariae*). Humans are the only reservoir for these species. Malaria in animals is caused by other species of plasmodia, and there is evidence that the four human plasmodia have cognate species in nonhuman primates from which they evolved.[1] Human infection is endemic in parts of Asia, Africa, Central and South America, Oceania, and some Caribbean islands.[2]

Louis M. Katz, MD, Vice President, Medical Affairs, Mississippi Valley Regional Blood Center, Davenport, Iowa

The Pathogen, Its Occurrence, and Global Impact

Malaria is a life-threatening infection, exacting its heaviest toll in sub-Saharan Africa. The World Health Organization (WHO) has estimated that there were 1,124,000 malaria deaths worldwide in 2001. Of those, 963,000 (85.7%) were in Africa. The human plasmodia are estimated to have caused 396 million cases of acute illness in 2001, with 86.4% in Africa, and are among the leading causes of death in young children.[3] Pregnant women are the most important adult risk group in most areas of the world where plasmodia are endemic. Malaria is an important cause of fetal wastage, low birthweight, and neonatal mortality.

Malaria retards development in developing countries with endemic and epidemic disease, costing African economies more than US$12 billion annually. WHO estimates that African gross domestic products are 32% smaller than predicted had malaria been eradicated in 1960.[4]

Malaria transmission is determined by the presence and abundance of susceptible female anopheline mosquitoes (the insect vector), whether the hosts they select for blood meals are infected, and whether the vector survives long enough after an infectious blood meal for the parasite to complete its sexual life cycle and for transmission to occur during a subsequent blood meal. The latter is mainly influenced by temperature and humidity.

Transmission is seen mainly in tropical (and, to a lesser extent, subtropical) areas of the developing world. In the past, malaria (*P. malariae* and *P. vivax*) was epidemic as far north as Finland.[5] *P. vivax* is the most widely distributed species and predominates in temperate areas where malaria is endemic. *P. falciparum* predominates in most tropical areas. *P. ovale* is uncommon and seen mostly in areas of sub-Saharan West Africa. *P. malariae* is relatively rare but distributed patchily worldwide.

High malaria transmission rates persist in areas of Papua-New Guinea, Brazil, Southeast Asia, and most of sub-Saharan

Africa. *P. falciparum* transmission is particularly intense in the tropics. Resistance of *P. falciparum* to chloroquine, other 4-aminoquinolines, and other antimalarial drugs has become widespread. Chloroquine-resistant *P. vivax* infection is an emerging problem in Indonesia, Papua-New Guinea, parts of Oceania, and Guyana.

Malaria is not rare in the United States. Figure 6-1 shows the number of cases of malaria diagnosed among civilians in this country from the early 1970s through 2000. During the last 20 years, between 1000 and 1500 cases have been seen annually, with over half in US residents in recent years. Table 6-1 displays the *Plasmodium* species and area of acquisition of almost 1400 imported cases of malaria recognized in the United States in 2000. Figure 6-2 displays the infecting species in reported cases in the United States during four periods since 1963. The recent increase of *P. falciparum* cases reflects patterns of travel to and immigration from areas where this species predominates. Local transmission (mosquito transmission apparently occurring in the United States) is very rare but is certainly possible given a reservoir of individuals with infection acquired in countries where the disease is endemic, the presence of

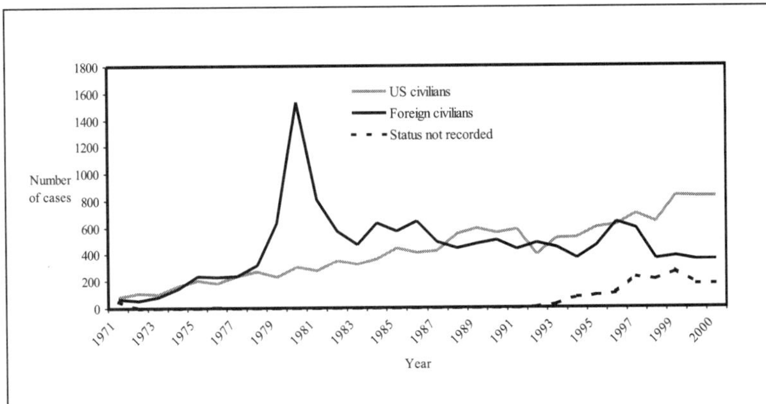

Figure 6-1. US malaria cases by country of origin 1971-2000 (excluding US military personnel). Adapted from Mungai et al[6] and the CDC.[7]

Table 6-1. Imported Malaria Cases by Region of Acquisition and *Plasmodium* Species—United States, 2000*

Region of Acquisition	*P. falciparum*	*P. vivax*	*P. malariae*	*P. ovale*	Unknown	Mixed	Total
Africa	528	92	40	31	85	7	783
Asia	17	176	11	1	33	0	238
Central America and Caribbean	22	147	8	0	22	1	200
North America	2	24	1	0	3	0	30
South America	9	41	3	0	4	0	57
Oceania	2	17	1	0	2	0	22
Europe and newly independent states	0	0	0	0	0	0	0
Unknown	29	24	2	0	12	1	68
Total	609	521	66	32	161	9	1398

*Adapted from the CDC.[7]

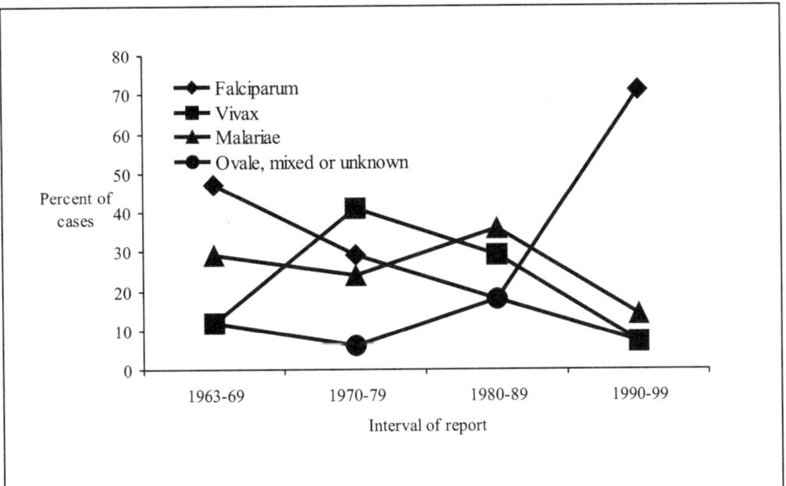

Figure 6-2. Species of *Plasmodium* causing transfusion-induced malaria in the United States by time interval of report. Adapted from Mungai et al.[6]

competent anopheline vectors, and appropriate environmental conditions for the maturation of the parasite. Only 17 cases of local transmission in 10 outbreaks were identified between 1992 and 1999, with two cases reported from Virginia in 2002.[8,9]

The Disease

Classic clinical malaria is characterized by periodic fever and rigors, sweats, splenomegaly, and hemolytic anemia; however, the manifestations at various times after infection, in semi-immune vs nonimmune hosts, and related to individual species are protean and the reader is directed to standard texts to appreciate the spectrum of the disease.[10,11] The four species can present with sufficiently similar symptoms so that they can be clinically indistinguishable. *P. vivax* and *P. ovale* infect relatively young red cells, whereas *P. malariae* infects relatively old cells. This limits the susceptible cellular population available to the parasite, and disease from these three species is not usually lethal.

Unrecognized or untreated *P. falciparum* malaria produces very severe illness in nonimmune persons, in part related to its ability to infect red cells of all ages, resulting in very high levels of parasitemia, and also to the propensity of parasitized red cells to cause microvascular obstruction. Cerebral malaria is the most dangerous manifestation of severe *P. falciparum* malaria. It is mediated by a complex set of interactions of parasitized red cells, platelets, white cells, cytokines, and the vascular endothelium of the central nervous system, resulting in cellular sequestration, vascular obstruction, and tissue hypoxia.[12]

The clinical presentation of malaria, particularly early after onset and before the fever can become periodic, is nonspecific and can be confused with many other causes of fever if clinicians fail to obtain sufficient history to recognize the possibility of exposure to plasmodia. Some important clinical points deserve emphasis.

Untreated malaria, especially *P. falciparum* in nonimmune hosts, can be lethal less than 24 hours after clinical onset. Symptoms common to all species include fever and chills, which can be accompanied by nonspecific manifestations such as headache, myalgias, arthralgias, weakness, vomiting, and diarrhea. Other clinical features include splenomegaly, anemia, thrombocytopenia, hypoglycemia, pulmonary or renal dysfunction, and neurologic changes. The clinical presentation can vary substantially depending on the infecting species, the level of parasitemia, and the overall and malaria-specific immune status of the patient. Infections caused by *P. falciparum* can rapidly progress to severe, fatal forms with central nervous system involvement (cerebral malaria), acute renal failure, severe anemia, or adult respiratory distress syndrome, particularly in aboriginal children and travelers who lack prior exposure and immunity to the parasite. *P. malariae* manifestations can include the nephrotic syndrome.

Although it is axiomatic among infectious diseases clinicians in this country that *P. falciparum* malaria is the cause of fever in potentially exposed individuals until it has been excluded, malaria may not be the only infection present in residents of areas where the disease is endemic or in travelers to them. Thus, even the presence of parasites on a blood smear does not confirm malaria as the sole source of a febrile illness in the appropriate epidemiologic setting. Also, the clinical presentation can be modified by partial treatment or the use of chemoprophylaxis. This renders the diagnosis more difficult, requiring a very high index of suspicion and repeated testing.

A detailed discussion of the treatment of malaria is beyond the scope of this chapter. Two points are of great importance, however, to both clinicians and transfusion medicine specialists. First, the increasing occurrence of resistance to formerly active drugs in wide areas of the world demands very careful attention to the possible source of malarial infection, whether vector-borne or induced. In the case of transfusion-induced malaria, this may require empiric therapy because the source of donor infection may not be immediately apparent (donors must be identified, located, and interviewed). Second, radical cure with primaquine of relapsing species (*P. vivax* and *P. ovale*) should not be needed in transfusion-induced infection because the hypnozoite source of relapse is not involved in the pathogenesis of infection.

Reasonable recommendations for optimal therapy have been published,[13] but clinicians unfamiliar with malaria therapy are strongly cautioned to consult with experienced physicians to provide optimal therapy.

Diagnosis

Historically, the diagnosis of clinical malaria has been based on clinical suspicion followed by microscopic demonstration of the parasite on stained films of peripheral blood.[14]

The sensitivity of examination of Giemsa-stained thick and thin blood smears under ideal circumstances is at a parasite level of around 50 parasites/µL of blood. However, under clinical conditions in the United Kingdom, a sensitivity of 500 parasites/µL (0.01% of red cells) was demonstrated.[15] Standard microscopy is technique dependent, requires significant investment in equipment and training, and requires continuous experience to maintain operator proficiency. To overcome some or all of these difficulties, several other techniques for the diagnosis of malaria are available or being developed. These include fluorescence microscopy, antigen detection using immunochromatographic techniques primarily, flow cytometry, and nucleic acid detection.

These alternate methods vary in sensitivity and specificity, the range of malarial species detected, ability to estimate parasite density, speed of reversion to negative after treatment, skill required for use, equipment needed, and cost per test.[16] The performance characteristics and possible utility of these methods in clinical applications are beyond the scope of this chapter but have been discussed elsewhere.[17] The potential use of these approaches for donor screening applications will be discussed below.

Life Cycle and Transmission Routes

The parasite life cycle is complex and is reviewed in general texts on infectious diseases and parasitology.[10,11] Plasmodia are transmitted in nature when the infected female anopheline mosquito injects sporozoites from her salivary glands under the skin during a blood meal. Sporozoites transmitted to the host by the mosquito travel via the bloodstream to the liver, where they invade liver cells. Sporozoites of all four human plasmodia mature into liver (exoerythrocytic) schizonts, but, in *P. vivax* and *P. ovale* infections, some also become dormant hypnozoites, the tissue reservoir for these relapsing malarias. Schizonts in the liver develop into 10,000 to 40,000 exoerythrocytic merozoites per infected hepatocyte; these merozoites are released into the blood, where each can infect a red cell. There, in the asexual red cell cycle, they mature through ring, trophozoite, and schizont stages into 8 to 30 (depending on the species) erythrocytic merozoites that lyse the infected cell after 2 to 3 days, at which time they can infect more red cells. The classic paroxysms of malarial fever coincide with the synchronous rupture of these infected red cells [at 48 hours for *P. falciparum*, *P. vivax*, and *P. ovale* infections (tertian malarias) and 72 hours for *P. malariae* (quartan malaria)].

The hypnozoites of *P. vivax* and *P. ovale* may remain dormant in the liver for months to years and then mature to tissue schizonts, repeating the asexual cycle. This causes either symptomatic relapse, or a primary clinical infection if the initial attack was suppressed by chemoprophylaxis that was not followed by radical cure using primaquine to kill the hypnozoites.

A few red cell parasites of each species will differentiate into the male and female gametocytes that are infectious to vector mosquitoes, are taken during a blood meal, and complete their sexual life cycle in the insect gut and salivary glands.

Virtually all malaria is transmitted by the natural mosquito cycle. There are, however, two other recognized modes of transmission—congenital and induced.

Congenital malaria from an infected mother occurs after transplacental transmission. Pregnancy may make women more susceptible to infection, with an increased parasitemia facilitating passage of parasites across the placenta.[18]

Induced malaria occurs when blood that contains merozoites is injected. Because this route does not transmit sporozoites, liver hypnozoites cannot develop during induced *P. vivax* and *P. ovale* infection and relapses do not occur. Needle-sharing drug use with infected blood-containing paraphernalia is an example of induced malaria. Induced *P. vivax* infection (fever therapy) was used as treatment for neurosyphilis before the availability of effective antibiotics. Up to six paroxysms of fever from 103 to 106 F would be observed before the administration of quinine to abort the attack. A Nobel Prize in medicine was awarded to Julius Von Wagner-Jauregg in 1928 for the concept. Controlled studies were never done, and published results suggested treatment response was unpredictable and of variable durability.[19] Use of induced malaria to treat *Borrelia burgdorferi* infection (Lyme disease) was recently suggested[20] and has been reported.[21] The same author has employed this approach to human immunodeficiency virus (HIV).[22] The practice is discouraged because of the absence of evidence of efficacy, the morbidity of clinical malaria, and the possibility of simultaneous transmission of other blood-borne infections.[23]

Allogeneic organ and marrow transplantation have been implicated in the induction of malaria in a number of case reports and a small series.[24-29] Whether these incidents result from residual red cells in the various grafts or from the persistence of plasmodia in other cells in the allograft is not clear.

Transfusion-transmitted malaria is a form of induced malaria. Transmission of malaria by the injection of blood from patients into healthy persons was demonstrated in 1884.[30] Woolsey reported transmission by fresh blood transfusion in 1911.[31] Transmission of malaria by stored blood was reported in 1941.[32]

Epidemiology of Transfusion-Induced Malaria

As with other transfusion-transmissible infections, the potential impact of transfusion-induced malaria is greater in developing nations than developed countries. Estimates of incidence in the countries of endemicity are confounded by lack of reporting and by preexisting infection in transfusion recipients. Although high-quality data on the incidence of clinical malaria after blood transfusion in the developing world are not available, some recent studies have examined the prevalence of parasitemia in blood donors in those areas and demonstrate very high risk.

A cross-sectional study[33] of 355 healthy blood donors during the rainy season in Cotonou, Benin used microscopic examination of blood smears. The results showed that 33.5% of donors were parasitemic and likely capable of transmitting the parasite via their blood donation. No relationship between the load of parasitized red cells and clinical malaria in the donors was observed. *P. falciparum* accounted for 96.6% of the donor infections. Another study[34] of 364 healthy blood donors in Nigeria screened for *P. falciparum* by microscopy showed that 4.1% were positive. In Benin City, Nigeria, blood smears for malaria parasites on donor blood demonstrated a prevalence of 40%, with *P. falciparum* the predominant species.[35] It should be remembered that estimates derived from blood smears in donors represent minimum potential donor rates because partial immunity in adult donors will often reduce parasitemia to below the threshold for detection on thick blood smears.

Data on the US incidence of transfusion-induced malaria have been recently and comprehensively reviewed.[6] The degree to which the data are affected by underrecognition and underreporting is not known. During the years 1963 to 1999, 93 cases were recognized and reported from 28 states. Between 0 and 9 cases were seen annually during that interval, with an incidence range estimated between 0 and 1.37 cases per million units of whole blood and red cells transfused. A peak seen from the late 1960s into the early 1970s was attributed to the return of military personnel from Vietnam and increasing emigration from Southeast Asia. A second peak in the late 1970s and early 1980s remains unexplained. From 1993 through 1998, a low, stable incidence between 0 and 0.18 case per million units has been maintained. The mortality from these cases was 11% (10 of 93 patients); six deaths were associated with *P. falciparum* infection. In 1999 and 2000, the most recent years for which data are available, no cases of transfusion-induced malaria were reported to the Centers for Disease Control and Prevention (CDC).[7,8] A single cryptic case in August 2001 may have been related to transfusion, but the donor investigation was incomplete (Parise M, CDC Malaria Branch, personal communication).

Species Involved in Transfusion

Historically, *P. malariae* has been most closely associated with transfusion-induced malaria, followed by *P. vivax* and *P. falciparum*. The association with *P. malariae* results from its long persistence in semi-immune infected individuals. During the 1970s, official reports from about 40 countries to WHO demonstrated an increasing incidence of *P. vivax* and *P. falciparum*, with a relative decline in the incidence of *P. malariae*.[36] Reports from individual countries and regions during these time frames showed substantial variation and call into question the precision of estimates derived from "officially" reporting countries.

In the United States, data from CDC surveillance show that *P. falciparum* became the predominant species in transfusion-induced malaria during the 1990s (Fig 6-2). This rise in cases caused by *P. falciparum* coincides with an increase in the proportion of transmission from immigrants from countries where malaria is endemic and a decline in the proportion of transmission from military personnel returning to the United States.

An important determinant of the ability of a blood donor to transmit malaria is the ability of the parasite to persist in the human host. With *P. vivax* and *P. ovale* infection, survival of hypnozoites can result in clinical relapse for up to 3 years, but substantially longer persistence is recognized, including the setting of transfusion transmission. As a result, transmission of *P. vivax* has been documented 27 years after the last recognizable exposure[37]; transmission of *P. ovale* was documented after 7 years.[38] *P. falciparum* infections generally die out within 12 to 18 months, but longer persistence has been documented, and transfusion transmission 13 years after potential exposure has been reported.[37] *P. malariae*, although lacking a hypnozoite liver stage, can persist in parasitized red cells in the face of strong humoral immunity for many years, resulting in clinical recrudescence after as long as 70 years and transfusion transmission even 53 years after infection.[39] Thus, one cannot prevent all cases of transfusion-induced malaria using donor history exclusions.

Implicated Components and Survival in Stored Components

Whole Blood and Red Blood Cell (RBC) units are the primary vectors of transfusion-induced malaria. Platelet and leukocyte transfusions contain variable numbers of red cells and have induced malaria.[40,41] There are data suggesting that merozoites can infect platelets, but the relevance of this finding to transfusion-induced malaria is unknown.[42] Frozen RBCs have also been implicated in transmission at the case report level,[43] and the parasites survive well in frozen blood.[44] Transmission by fresh plasma has been described,[45] but in the recent US experience,[6] in the patients for whom a component was implicated, 94% of those components were whole blood or red cells and 6% were platelets.

Induction of malaria for the treatment of neurosyphilis allowed the investigation of the survival of malaria in blood. In 92 cases, the infectivity of *P. vivax* declined after 3 days in storage,[46] but infectivity persisted at 8 days. In 32 cases of induced malaria, the addition of 3% to 4% dextrose was associated with transmission of *P. vivax* after 10 days and *P. falciparum* after 21 days of storage.[47] All human malarial parasites remain viable in stored blood for over a week, and studies from the 1960s demonstrate longer survival (>10 days) with dextrose-containing anticoagulants.[48-50] Data on the duration of storage of implicated components in US cases of transfusion-induced malaria is not routinely collected (Parise M, CDC Malaria Branch, personal communication). Likewise, few data exist describing the survival of plasmodia in currently used blood bags with contemporary anticoagulants, although one study suggested that the addition of adenine (substituting CPD-A for CPD) diminished the viability of *P. falciparum*.[51]

US donors can be implicated in a case of transfusion-induced malaria if they have a positive blood smear, reactive malaria serology, or positive polymerase chain reaction (PCR), or if they are the sole donor to a recipient with transfusion-induced malaria.[7] Malaria surveillance by the CDC demonstrates that, except for the period of greatest immigration from Southeast Asia in the late 1970s and early 1980s, total malaria cases in the United States have been almost evenly divided among US and foreign nationals.[7] During the late 1990s, the proportion among US citizens appeared to be increasing. In

2000, 70% of US civilian malaria cases occurred in US residents. When considering only the donors of components implicated in transfusion-induced malaria cases from 1963 to 1999, 59% of the implicated donors whose country of origin could be ascertained were foreign-born. Among donors implicated in 1990 to 1999, 10/12 (83%) were foreign-born.[6] Potential areas from which infection was acquired could be determined for 64 of the 91 implicated donors. Thirty-one were from sub-Saharan Africa, 21 from south and southeast Asia, four from southern Europe and the Mediterranean, four from Mexico, three from the rest of the Americas, and one had been in more than one area.

Clinical Transfusion-Induced Malaria

Recognition of transfusion-related malaria is dependent on a high index of suspicion in febrile transfusion recipients. The incubation period for transfusion-induced malaria is dependent on the numbers of parasites infused, the *Plasmodium* species, and probably the susceptibility of the host. With *P. falciparum* and *P. vivax* malaria, this is from 1 week to 1 month, but with *P. malariae*, it may be measured in months.[52] Longer incubation periods may make the association with transfusion difficult to recognize or establish. Historically, *P. malariae* is associated with the longest incubation (mean 57 days), followed by *P. vivax* (20 days) and *P. falciparum* (16 days).[53] The maximum incubations in this study were 109, 30, and 29 days, respectively, for the three species. In the more recent US series,[6] the mean values were very similar (50, 20, and 17 days for the three species, respectively), but ranges were not provided to identify the extreme outliers. The interval from clinical onset to diagnosis in these cases was 1 to 180 days (median 10). These data demonstrate that the diagnosis must be considered in any patient with a compatible clinical syndrome who was transfused within a period of even longer than 3 months.

Fever is the clinical hallmark of transfusion-induced malaria, but the classic periodic fevers of tertian and quartan malaria are unusual. Additional nonspecific symptoms include malaise, nausea, vomiting, and abdominal discomfort.[54] Obviously, among a population of patients ill enough to require transfusions, there is considerable overlap of these symptoms with those of the underlying illnesses and the complications of hospitalization, including nosocomial infection. This is likely to be associated with a delay in consideration of the diagnosis, particularly in countries where the disease is not endemic and induced malaria is rare, eg, the United States. This may be compounded by the increasing reliance on automated hematology analyzers that have reduced the number of peripheral blood smears examined by experienced microscopists.

Eleven percent of the cases of transfusion-induced malaria in the United States from 1963 to 1999 were fatal. Six were *P. falciparum* and two each were *P. vivax* and *P. malariae*.[6] This is much higher than the current mortality of vector-associated malaria in the United States. Six of 1402 (0.43%) cases recorded in 2000 were fatal, 3/873 among US civilians and military, and 3/354 in foreigners (status was not recorded in 175).[7] One can speculate that the higher apparent mortality in transfusion-induced cases, compared with recent vector-borne malaria, is attributable to delay in consideration and diagnosis of induced cases, lack of immunity in patients with induced malaria, and confounding by the clinical manifestations of the underlying condition(s) requiring transfusion.

Prevention of Transfusion-Induced Malaria

Prevention of transfusion-induced malaria has depended primarily on the elicitation of a history of risk for plasmodium infection from prospective donors. This includes a history of residence in or travel to regions where the disease is considered endemic, generally using CDC or WHO lists of areas with risk of transmission.[55,56]

The criteria for identifying at-risk donors in the United States have evolved over time with the development of regulations from the Food and Drug Administration (FDA) and voluntary standards from the American Association of Blood Banks. The general evolution of malaria criteria can be summarized briefly. During the 1950s and 1960s, donors were initially required to be free of diseases transmissible by transfusion, and then explicit listing of freedom from malaria and syphilis were added to the donor interview. During the 1970s, the requirements were amended to include specific time frames for temporary deferral, based on travel to or resident status in areas of endemicity: 1 year for travelers and 3 years for residents. Use of antimalarial chemoprophylaxis by travelers resulted in a 3-year deferral, compared with 1 year for travel without treatment, on the assumption that it could modify the clinical evolution of malaria and result in unrecognized, prolonged infection of donors. A 3-year deferral for prospective donors treated for malaria was included. In 1994, the longer deferrals for donors who were residents of regions where malaria was not endemic traveling to areas where it was endemic, and for those who had taken chemoprophylaxis, were rescinded. A uniform 1-year time frame was allowed for these groups of donors.

The most current blood donor historical screening criteria are codified in draft guidance from the FDA[57]:

- Prospective donors with a history of malaria are deferred for 3 years after becoming asymptomatic.
- Immigrants, refugees, and citizens from countries where malaria is considered endemic by the CDC Malaria Branch are deferred for 3 years after their departure, provided they have been free of otherwise unexplained symptoms suggestive of malaria.
- Travelers from areas where malaria is not endemic to areas where it is endemic can be accepted as blood donors 12 months after their departure from the area of endemicity, provided they have been free of otherwise unexplained symptoms suggestive of malaria, regardless of receipt of antimalarial chemoprophylaxis.

- An exception is made for visitors to certain areas in the Republic of Korea, who are deferred for 2 years, related to the identification of *P. vivax* malaria with a prolonged incubation period in this temperate region.[58]

Review of data on US transfusion-induced malaria[6] suggests that complete elicitation of an appropriate donor history using these deferral criteria would have resulted in the exclusion of 37/60 (62%) of the implicated donors for whom adequate information was available. Likewise, 30/48 (62%) should have been deferred by using the criteria extant at the time they transmitted the infection. Of the remaining donors from whom responses to the interview questions were appropriately elicited, 15/23 (65%) were infected with *P. malariae*, and because of its long persistence in asymptomatic infections, no practical historical deferral would be expected to be effective. Recognizing these failures of the interview process, the Uniform Donor History Task Force of the AABB has recommended changing the donor screening method to one that does not depend on the prospective donors' understanding of where in the world malaria is endemic. To accomplish this, the task force proposes to ask donors "In the past 3 years, have you been outside the United States and Canada?" with affirmative answers followed up by more specific interviewing regarding where the donor has been for comparison against countries with endemic malaria (Fridey J, AABB Uniform Donor History Questionnaire Task Force, personal communication).

An audiovisual touch screen computer-assisted donor interview using the AABB Uniform Donor History Questionnaire at a US blood center was unable to reduce travel-related postdonation information reports leading to malaria deferrals, despite eliciting significantly more risk behaviors relevant to HIV infection, so it is unclear what elements an improved interview process would require to more fully elicit malaria risk.[59]

Obviously, malaria-endemic countries cannot use residential criteria and maintain a robust blood supply. In malaria-free regions, the loss of safe donors due to the low positive predictive value of geographic exclusions results in the deferral of a large number of donors without malaria. Based on extrapolation of a survey of US independent community blood centers in 1998, it was estimated that travel and residence criteria for blood donation resulted in the deferral of approximately 50,000 blood donors nationwide annually (Bianco C, America's Blood Centers, personal communication). Accordingly, laboratory methods of malaria detection to prevent transmission have been considered for use in all settings, regardless of endemicity.

It is likely that none of the approaches for asymptomatic donors described will be completely effective as donor screens, even in the most experienced hands, because inoculation of mice with a single parasite can induce malaria[60] and human malaria can be transmitted by inoculating not more than 10 parasites of *P. vivax*.[61] If this can be generalized to a unit of RBCs, it corresponds to a parasite density around 0.00004 parasites/µL of blood, well below the sensitivity of even PCR and far lower than that of microscopy or antigen detection.

The utility of a putative donor-screening test for malaria will vary according to its performance characteristics and the expected prevalence of infection in asymptomatic donors. As noted above, the latter will be very high in areas of extreme endemicity, but very low in US blood donors, on the basis of the frequency of transfusion-induced malaria. Tests for malaria are developed for clinical diagnostic indications where pretest probabilities are high, not for asymptomatic donor screening, so their performance characteristics in low-prevalence populations such as US blood donors is generally unknown. Therefore, deployment of screening assays would, require careful consideration of what set of donors should be tested. Universal screening in areas of high malaria prevalence may be justified, whereas selection for testing of only the subset of asymptomatic prospective donors who have apparent risk due to travel or residence in regions where malaria is endemic may be optimal in countries with no endemicity.

Thick and thin blood films prepared with Giemsa or Wright's stains remain the preferred clinical diagnostic tests worldwide. In addition to providing diagnostic information, a blood smear allows identification of parasite species and semiquantitation of parasitemia, which correlate with the severity of disease and, in some cases, influence therapy. Blood smears involve microscopic examination of slides of blood from a finger or earlobe stick or from venipuncture. The former are preferred, being capillary rich and a better source of parasitized red cells.[62] Blood film interpretation is very experience-dependent. It requires substantial supplies and fragile equipment and may take 1 hour or more for preparation and examination of the slides. Although in the most experienced hands, sensitivities of 5 to 50 parasites/μL can be attained, in routine use, a thick blood smear may have a sensitivity of only 500 parasites/μL of red cells.[15] Only 25% of implicated donors in the US series of cases were smear positive.[6] As a result of these concerns, one must consider blood smears unsuitable for routine use in blood collection facilities in either the developing or developed world.

Fluorescence microscopy diagnostic techniques, using acridine orange and other dyes, have been developed to enhance the detection of plasmodia for diagnostic applications.[16] They are rapid, but they require sophisticated equipment; they can be nonspecific; and sensitivity for low level parasitemia, as would be found in asymptomatic blood donors, appears to be inferior to standard examination of blood smears.[63] They have not been evaluated in donor screening applications and do not seem applicable to routine screening of prospective donors.

P. falciparum antigen detection assays are being developed for diagnostic indications. Malaria antigens suitable for rapid detection assays include histidine-rich protein 2 (HRP-2), plasmodium lactate dehydrogenase (pLDH), and aldolase. They can be detected using a variety of immunochromatographic techniques and, in general, have parasite sensitivities of >100 parasites/μL,[16] which is probably superior to the results obtained by most microscopists outside expert laboratories. In addition, they are available on dipsticks that require minimal expertise and can be completed in about 20 minutes. Limitations as blood donor screens include inadequate sensitivity to prevent many cases of transfusion-induced malaria from asymptomatic donors with low parasite densities and variable sensitivity for non-*P. falciparum* human plasmodia. Despite these limitations, these assays may find utility in areas with endemic malaria as "low-technology" means to exclude many parasitemic donors.

PCR is more sensitive and specific than other techniques.[64] It is a technically complex procedure that is not currently appropriate for clinical use in the field but has been considered for blood donor screening because of its exquisite specificity and sensitivity. PCR applied to blood donors in Vietnam demonstrated an improved sensitivity compared with peripheral blood smears, detecting 19/30 donors with low-level parasitemia compared to 4/30 by smear.[65] An assay for *P. falciparum* applied to potential donors in Spain at risk for malaria has a sensitivity of between 0.004 and 0.04 parasite/µL and detected smear-negative, presumptively infectious, donors.[66] Although this sensitivity is between 100 and 1000 times better than microscopy in expert hands, it represents 1000 to 10,000 parasites in 250 mL of red cells, so it would not provide complete protection against transfusion-induced malaria. Given the low incidence, the cost per transfusion-induced malaria infection averted would be millions of dollars in countries where malaria is not endemic.[67] Selective use for those with an appropriate travel or residence history is unlikely to salvage donors because the estimated sensitivity of PCR is not great enough to exclude infection.

Substantial experience has been gained using malaria antibody detection to screen donors at risk for prior malaria infection and for confirmation of a smear-negative, asymptomatic donor as the probable source of a transfusion-induced case.[68] An antibody assay makes particular sense to qualify prospective donors with a history of travel to or residence in countries of endemicity because antibody tests turn positive within a few weeks of infection. The French defer donors returning from countries where malaria is endemic for 4 months and screen donors 4 months to 3 years following return with an indirect immunofluorescent antibody assay. No transfusion-induced malaria has been reported since the beginning of mandatory reporting of transfusion complications in 1994.[69] Using a risk-based application of antibody assays, British investigators have estimated "the ability to safely retrieve 40,000 RBC units currently discarded each year in Great Britain."[70] In the United States, 58/59 (98%) of implicated donors to transfusion-induced cases were seropositive using an immunofluorescence assay.[6]

The disadvantages of antibody assays are several. A true positive antibody assay may reflect not only current clinical or subclinical malaria, but also remote, long-resolved, or effectively treated infection. The latter situations may result in deferral of noninfectious donors. This is a particular disincentive in countries of endemicity, where such donor loss would be substantial. Poorly characterized cross-reactivity for specific non-*P. falciparum* species (many antigen preparations are derived from *P. falciparum*) may result in missing infections with these species. Nonspecificity of antibody assays may also result in deferral of otherwise acceptable donors, although methods to reduce this issue are being studied.[71] Finally, immunofluorescent studies are not generally considered to be useful for large-volume screening in the United States. Enzyme-linked immunoassay technology does exist, but performance characteristics have not been ideal,[69] and, to the author's knowledge, there are no candidate assays under review by the US FDA for approval in donor screening.

In the United States, precedent for selective serologic screening of blood donors is found in the use of cytomegalovirus (CMV) antibody only for those units ordered for patients recognized to be at risk for transfusion-associated CMV infection. To the degree malaria serology can be used to save donors from prolonged deferral, this strategy is attractive.

The high prevalence of parasitemia in partially immune prospective donors from areas with high malaria endemicity can compromise the availability of blood donors. Some have undertaken donor treatment with antimalarial chemoprophylaxis, or treatment of blood recipients with therapeutic courses of antimalarial drugs with substantial success.[52] Administration of therapeutic courses of antimalarial drugs to both blood donors and blood recipients was used with apparent success by the Australians in the Pacific theatre during World War II, and similar results have been obtained in West Africa and Vietnam.[52] These approaches using contemporary donors in countries of endemicity would need to be informed by local patterns of sensitivity of plasmodia to available medications.

The addition of chloroquine to anticoagulant used to prepare components has been suggested,[72] based on pharmacokinetic considerations that allow supratherapeutic exposure of the parasites to the medication that would be adequate to overcome antimalarial resistance, with minimal exposure of the recipient. The author is not aware of clinical data validating this approach.

Pathogen Reduction Technology

In order to further reduce the residual risk of known pathogens in blood components, and to preempt emerging and future pathogens, several companies are developing pathogen reduction systems. Those farthest along in development target nucleic acids (DNA and RNA) of viruses, bacteria, fungi, and parasites to abolish their capacity to replicate. The processes being studied must be robust in the spectrum of target microorganisms and preserve the function of the component. In-vitro data have demonstrated excellent activity against the commonly recognized organisms of relevance to transfusion.[73] There is preliminary work suggesting that the three approaches that have reached advanced stages of development will inactivate substantial levels of malaria parasites. None of these systems is available in the United States yet, pending completion of adequate clinical trials and adequate demonstration of their safety to the FDA.

Amotosalen (formerly S59) is a psoralen added to platelets or plasma that are then irradiated using ultraviolet (UV) light. The process results in covalent cross-linking of RNA and DNA strands, inhibiting nucleic acid replication. Limited studies using apheresis platelet units inoculated with red cells infected with *P. falciparum* demonstrate inactivation to below the limit of detection of parasites after inoculation with 4×10^6 (8 - 11% parasitized) cells/mL of component.[74]

Red cells absorb the UV light used to activate psoralens, so they are not effective in this product. S303 is a frangible anchor linker effector (FRALE) that cross-links nucleic acids in a radiation-independent fashion being developed to allow pathogen reduction of red cells. This compound has been shown to inactivate approximately 10^7 *P. falciparum* in inoculated full RBC units (Dupuis K, Cerus Corp, personal communication).

Inactines are small water-soluble compounds with high selectivity for nucleic acids that produce strand breaks and inhibit replication. One of these, PEN 110, is undergoing clinical development for pathogen reduction in red cells. At concentrations of 0.01 to 0.1%, PEN 110 was able to inactivate *P. falciparum* in human red cells.[75]

Riboflavin, vitamin B2, intercalates between the bases in RNA and DNA. When exposed to visible or UV light, it induces strand breaks and covalent adducts in the nucleic acid, inhibiting replication. It is being developed for pathogen reduction of plasma, platelets, and red cells. In experiments using *P. falciparum* added to red cells to create a 6% to 13% parasitemia, complete inactivation was observed with the use of 500 mM of riboflavin and 60 minutes of illumination with visible light.[76]

An effective vaccine would be a stunning public health accomplishment, given the morbidity and mortality of malaria in the developing world. The subjects of malaria immunity and vaccinology are too broad for this chapter, but effective immunization against malaria could enhance the safety of blood in the developing world and offer protection to blood donors traveling to regions of endemicity. A *P. falciparum* candidate targeted at the development of humoral immunity to the pre-erythrocytic phase of the parasite life cycle has demonstrated 71% protective efficacy after 2 months in Gambia, but this was no longer measurable by the end of the 15-week follow-up period.[77] Animal models of vaccines designed to stimulate cell-mediated immunity to pre-erythrocytic parasites using a DNA vaccine followed by a recombinant vaccinia vector encoding malarial proteins are promising,[78] and field trials will be performed. Multiple other vaccine initiatives are in progress, but as a strategy for the prevention of transfusion-induced infection, all are many years off.

Summary

Malaria remains a rare but serious complication of transfusion in much of the world. Control continues to rely primarily on effective elicitation and interpretation of the donors' residence and travel histories. The current approach to prevention is highly effective, but errors in donor history screening as currently practiced permit a substantial proportion of the transfusion-induced cases seen in the United States and also result in the deferral of thousands of uninfected donors during an era of tight blood supplies. Of the available methods to improve outcomes, screening of high-risk donors with serology holds promise to reduce unneeded donor deferrals but would require approval and implementation of serologic tests with better performance characteristics than are currently available. The ultimate elimination of transfusion-induced malaria will likely require pathogen reduction systems.

References

1. Coatney GR, Collins WE, Warren M, et al. The primate malarias. Washington, DC: US Government Printing Office,1971:1-340.

2. Malaria. In: Chin J, ed. Control of communicable diseases manual. 17th ed. Washington, DC: American Public Health Association, 2000: 310-23.
3. World Health Organization. The world health report. Geneva, Switzerland: World Health Organization, 2002. [Available at www.who.int/whr/2002/en/.]
4. World Health Organization. Report of the Commission on Macroeconomics and Health of the World Health Organization. Geneva, Switzerland: World Health Organization, 2002.
5. Rietveld A. Frequently asked questions about malaria. [Available at http://mosquito.who.int/cgi-bin/rbm/dhome_rbm.jsp.]
6. Mungai M, Tegtmaier G, Chamberland M, et al. Transfusion-transmitted malaria in the United States from 1963 through 1999. N Engl J Med 2001;344:1973-8.
7. Centers for Disease Control and Prevention. Malaria surveillance—United States, 2000. MMWR Morb Mortal Wkly Rep 2002;51(No. SS-5):9-21.
8. Centers for Disease Control and Prevention. Malaria surveillance—United States, 1999. MMWR Morb Mortal Wkly Rep 2002;51(No. SS-1):15-28.
9. Centers for Disease Control and Prevention. Local transmission of *Plasmodium vivax* malaria—Virginia, 2002. MMWR Morb Mortal Wkly Rep 2002;51:921-3.
10. Krogstad DJ. Plasmodium species (malaria). In: Mandell GL, Bennett JE, Dolin R, eds. Principles and practice of infectious diseases. Philadelphia: Churchill-Livingstone, 2000:2817-31.
11. Strickland GT. Malaria. In: Strickland GT, ed. Hunter's tropical medicine. Philadelphia: WB Saunders, 1991:586-617.
12. Lou J, Lucas R, Grau GE. Pathogenesis of cerebral malaria: Recent experimental data and possible applications for humans. Clin Microbiol Rev 2001;14(4):810-20.
13. Advice for travelers. Treatment for parasitic infections. Med Lett Drugs Ther 2002;44(1128):33-8.
14. Warhurst DC, Williams JE. Laboratory diagnosis of malaria. J Clin Pathol 1996;49:533-8.
15. Milne L, Chiodini PL, Warhurst, DC. Accuracy of routine laboratory diagnosis of malaria in the United Kingdom. J Clin Pathol 1994;47: 740-2.
16. Moody A. Rapid diagnostic tests for malaria. Clin Microbiol Rev 2002;15(1):66-78.
17. New perspective, malaria diagnosis: Report of a joint WHO/USAID informal consultation. Geneva, Switzerland: World Health Organization, 2000. [Available at www.who.int/tdr/publications/publications/pdf/malaria_diagnosis.pdf.]
18. Brabin BJ. An analysis of malaria in pregnancy in Africa. Bull World Health Organ 1983;61:1005-16.

19. Mayne B. A review of selected papers contributing to the progress of malaria therapy during the past year. South Med J 1936;29:755-7.
20. Heimlich HJ. Should we try malariotherapy for Lyme disease? (letter). N Engl J Med 1990;322:1234-5.
21. Centers for Disease Control and Prevention. Imported malaria associated with malariotherapy of Lyme disease—New Jersey. MMWR Morb Mortal Wkly Rep 1990;39(48):873-5.
22. Heimlich HJ, Chen XP, Xiao BQ, et al. Malariotherapy for HIV patients. Mech Ageing Dev 1997;93(1-3):79-85.
23. Centers for Disease Control and Prevention. Update: Self-induced malaria associated with malariotherapy for Lyme disease—Texas. MMWR Morb Mortal Wkly Rep 1991;40(39):665-6.
24. Lefavour GS, Pierce JC, Frame JD. Renal transplant associated malaria. JAMA 1980;244(16):1820-1.
25. Dharmasena F, Gordon-Smith EC. Transmission of malaria by bone marrow transplantation (letter). Transplant 1986;42(2):228.
26. Crafa F, Gugenheim J, Fabiani P, et al. Possible transmission of malaria by liver transplantation. Transplant Proc 1991;23(5):2664.
27. Babinet J, Gay F, Bustos D, et al. Transmission of *Plasmodium falciparum* by heart transplant. Br Med J 1991;303:1515-6.
28. Turkmen A, Sever MS, Ecder T, et al. Posttransplant malaria. Transplantation 1996;62:1521-3.
29. Raina V, Sharma A, Gujral S, et al. *Plasmodium vivax* causing pancytopenia after allogeneic blood stem cell transplantation in CML. Bone Marrow Transplant 1998;22:205-6.
30. Gerhardt C. Ueber intermittens-impfungen. Z Klin Med 1884; 7:372.
31. Woolsey G. Transfusion for pernicious anemia: Two cases. Ann Surg 1911;53:132-4.
32. Gordon EF. Accidental transmission of malaria through administration of stored blood. JAMA 1941;116:1200.
33. Kinde-Gazard, Oke J, Gnahoui I, Massougbodji A. The risk of malaria transmission by blood transfusion at Cotonou, Benin. Sante 2000; 10(6):389-92.
34. Chikwem JO, Mohammed I, Okara GC, et al. Prevalence of transmissible blood infections among blood donors at the University of Maiducuri Teaching Hospital, Maiduguri, Nigeria. East Afr Med J 1997;74(4):213-6.
35. Ibhanesebhor SE, Otobo ES, Ladipo OA. Prevalence of malaria parasitaemia in transfused donor blood in Benin City, Nigeria. Ann Trop Paediatr 1996;16(2):93-5.
36. Bruce-Chwatt LJ. Transfusion malaria revisited. Trop Dis Bull 1982; 79(10):827-40.
37. Besson P, Robert JF, Reviron J. A propos de deux observations du paludisme transfusionnel: Essai de prévention associant un test d'immunofluorescence indirecte aux critères de sélection clinique. Rev Fr Transfus Immunohématol 1976;19:369-73.

38. Nahlen BL, Lobel HO, Cannon SE, et al. Reassessment of blood donor selection criteria for United States travelers to malarious areas. Transfusion 1991;31:798-804.
39. Guazzi M, Grazi S. A relapse of quartan malaria after 53 years latency. Trop Dis Bull 1964;61:11-12.
40. Garfield MD, Ershler WB, Maki DG. Malaria transmission by platelet concentrate transfusion. JAMA 1978;240:2285-6.
41. Dover AS, Guinee VF. Malaria transmission by leukocyte component therapy. JAMA 1971;217:1701-2.
42. Fajardo LF, Tallent C. Malarial parasites with human platelets. JAMA 1974;229:1205-7.
43. Najem GR, Sulzer AJ. Transfusion-induced malaria from an asymptomatic carrier. Transfusion 1976;16:473-6.
44. Kark JA. Malaria transmitted by blood transfusion. In: Tabor E, ed. Infectious complications of blood transfusion. New York: Academic Press, 1982:93-126.
45. Lazner EL, Newhouser LR. Studies on the transmissibility of malaria by plasma transfusions. Am J Med Sci 1943;206:141-6.
46. Antchelevitch WD. Transfusion von konserviertem malarikerblut. Folia Haematologia 1937;57:406-16.
47. Boventer K. The behaviour of malaria parasites in preserved blood. Trop Dis Bull 1949;46:799.
48. Duhanina NN, Zukova TA. Transmission of malaria by blood transfusion: An epidemiological study in the USSR. Bull World Health Organ 1965;33:853-6.
49. Carrescia PM. Malaria da trasfusione: Possibilita di profilassi. Riv Malariol 1960;39:209-20.
50. Morcos WM. Observations morphologiques de divers stades de *Plasmodium vivax* et de *Plasmodium malariae* dans le sang conserve à froid pour transfusion. Riv Malariol 1961;40:41-50.
51. Whaun JM, Webster HK. Altered purine metabolism in citrate-adenine stored blood: Implications for continuous in vitro *P. falciparum* culture. Clin Res 1981;29:352A.
52. Bruce-Chwatt L. Transfusion malaria. Bull World Health Organ 1974; 50:337-46.
53. Dover AS, Schultz MG. Transfusion-induced malaria. Transfusion 1971;11:353-7.
54. Bruce-Chwatt LJ. Transfusion malaria revisited. Trop Dis Bull 1982;79: 827-40.
55. Centers for Disease Control and Prevention. Health information for the international traveler 2001-2002. Atlanta, GA: US Department of Health and Human Services, Public Health Service, 2001.
56. World Health Organization. International travel and health. Malaria. [Available at: http://www.who.int/ith/chapter07_01.html.]
57. Food and Drug Administration. Draft guidance for industry: recommendations for donor questioning regarding possible exposure to malaria. (June 8, 2000) Rockville, MD: CBER Office of Communication,

Training, and Manufacturers Assistance, 2000. [Available at http://www.fda.gov/cber/gdlns/malaria.pdf.]

58. Fridey JL, ed. Standards for blood banks and transfusion services. 22nd ed. Bethesda, MD: American Association of Blood Banks, 2003: 72.
59. Katz LM. The computer assisted donor interview: A status report. Presented at the annual meeting of America's Blood Centers. Washington, DC, February 27, 2003.
60. Said A, Timperman G, Wery M. Effect of maintaining a strain of *Plasmodium berghei Anka* on gametogenesis. Ann Soc Belg Med Trop 1986;66:123-31.
61. Boyd MF. Epidemiology of malaria. In: Boyd MF, ed. Malariology. Philadelphia: WB Saunders, 1949;1:551-608.
62. Hommel M. Diagnostic methods in malaria. In: Gilles HM, Warrel DA, eds. Bruce-Chwatt's essential malariology. 3rd ed. London, UK: Hodder Arnold, 1993:35-58.
63. Wongsrichanalai C, Pornsilapatip J, Namsiriponpun V, et al. Acridine orange fluorescent microscopy and the detection of malaria in populations with low-density parasitemia. Am J Trop Med Hyg 1991;44: 17-20.
64. Snounou G, Viriyakosol S, Jarra W, et al. Identification of the four human malaria parasite species in field samples by the polymerase chain reaction and detection of a high prevalence of mixed infections. Mol Biochem Parasitol 1993;58:283-92.
65. Vu TT, Tran VB, Phan NT, et al. Screening donor blood for malaria by polymerase chain reaction. Trans R Soc Trop Med Hyg 1995;89:44-7.
66. Benito A, Rubio JM. Usefulness of semi-nested polymerase chain reaction for screening blood donors at risk for malaria in Spain (letter). Emerg Infect Dis 2001;7:1068.
67. Handscheid T, Valadas E, Grobusch MP. Polymerase chain reaction for screening blood donors at risk for malaria: Safe and useful? (letter) Emerg Infect Dis 2002;8:872.
68. Poole F. Antigen/antibody testing for malaria. Presented at the FDA Blood Products Advisory Committee meeting, Bethesda, MD, September 16, 1999. [Available at http://www.fda.gov/ohrms/dockets/ac/99/transcpt/3548t1.rtf.]
69. Silvie O, Thellier M, Rosenheim M, et al. Potential value of *Plasmodium falciparum*-associated antigen and antibody detection for screening blood donors to prevent transfusion-transmitted malaria. Transfusion 2002;42:357-62.
70. Chiodini PL, Hartley S, Hewitt PE, et al. Evaluation of a malaria antibody ELISA and its value in reducing potential wastage of red cell donations from blood donors exposed to malaria, with a note on a case of transfusion-transmitted malaria. Vox Sang 1997;73:143-8.
71. Soullie B, Soler C, Gerome P, et al. Specificity of immunofluorescent methods detecting malarial antibodies: Comparative study in the screening of blood donations. Transfus Clin Biol 2002;9:297-300.

72. White NJ. Chloroquine for donated blood? Lancet 1987;1(8524): 100-1.
73. Yun Y, Snyder EL. Safety of the blood supply: Role of pathogen reduction. Blood Rev 2003;17:111-22.
74. Dupuis K, Alfonso R, Labaied M, et al. The Intercept blood system for platelets inactivates *Plasmodium falciparum* (abstract). Transfusion 2002;42(Suppl):93S.
75. Zavizion B, Jorge MM, Pereira TN, et al. The Inactine PEN 110 chemistry eradicates the parasites that cause Chagas' disease, malaria and babesiosis. Vox Sang 2002;83(Suppl 2):118.
76. Lippert L, Watson R, Doane S, et al. Inactivation of *P. falciparum* by riboflavin and light. Vox Sang 2002;83(Suppl 2):163.
77. Ridley RG. Medical need, scientific opportunity and the drive for antimalarial drugs. Nature 2002;415:686-93.
78. Van Vugt M, Looareesuwan S, Wilairatana P, et al. Artemether-lumefantrine for the treatment of multidrug-resistant falciparum malaria. Trans R Soc Trop Med Hyg 2000;94:545-8.

In: Brecher ME, ed.
Bacterial and Parasitic Contamination of Blood Components
Bethesda, MD: AABB Press, 2003

7

Transmission of *T. cruzi* Infection by Blood Transfusion

IRA A. SHULMAN, MD

BLOOD COMPONENTS COLLECTED IN THE United States (US) may contain *Trypanosoma cruzi*, the parasite that causes Chagas' disease. Presently, in some communities (such as East Los Angeles), as many as one in every 1000 eligible blood donors has serologic evidence of *T. cruzi* infection, and perhaps over half of these individuals have intermittent parasitemia. The risk of transfusion-transmitted *T. cruzi* infection in the US, while small, ap-

Ira A. Shulman, MD, Associate Director, Laboratories/Director, Transfusion Medicine, Los Angeles County/University of Southern California Medical Center, Los Angeles, California

pears to be greatest for platelets, which are currently not subjected to heat or chemical treatment to inactivate infectious agents.

Trypanosoma cruzi Disease and Epidemiology

Chagas' disease is caused by the protozoan hemoflagellate *T. cruzi*,[1] which is endemic in the Western Hemisphere in rural areas of South America, Central America, and Mexico. It is usually transmitted to humans by the bite of an infected reduviid bug, although other mechanisms also exist. Reduviid bugs live in the burrows or nests of wild animals, and in dark, sheltered areas of human homes. They are frequently found to inhabit mud/adobe houses in Latin America. An estimated 16 to 18 million persons in Latin America are infected, and up to 25% of the total population of South and Central America is at risk.[1-4] An interesting time line of key events regarding Chagas' disease can be found at the World Health Organization web site at http://www.who. int/ctd/chagas/dates.htm.

In general, soon after an infected reduviid bug bites a human, the bug defecates feces that contain parasites.[3,4] The parasites can then pass through the site of the bite or be transferred to a mucous membrane if the bite is scratched or rubbed and the eyes or mouth are subsequently touched.[1] Humans come into contact with infected bugs if their homes are in an area where the disease is endemic and if the homes are constructed out of materials that can provide a suitable habitat, including thatched or tiled roofs and mud or stick walls. Vigorous efforts are being taken through the Southern Cone Initiative (http://www.who.int/ctd/chagas/epidemio.htm) to eliminate the chief regional vector of Chagas' disease in order to interrupt disease transmission in countries where it is endemic. See Table 7-1.[5,6]

Acute infection with *T. cruzi* is generally seen in children and can cause inflammation at the site of an insect bite or contaminated mucous membrane. Nonspecific or flu-like symptoms may be seen after an incubation period of one to several weeks. Symptoms usually resolve spontaneously in 4 to 8

Table 7-1. Human Infection by *Trypanosoma cruzi* and Reduction of Incidence*

Country	Age Group (Years)	Infection in 1983 (Rates × 100)	Infection in 1999 (Rates × 100)	Reduction of Incidence (%)
Argentina	18	4.5	1.2	85.0
Brazil	7-14	18.5	0.17	96.0
Bolivia	1-4	33.9	ND	ND
Chile	0-10	5.4	0.14	99.0
Paraguay	18	9.3	3.9	60.0
Uruguay	6-12	2.5	0.06	99.0

*Data from the Southern Cone Initiative.

weeks. The vast majority (>90%) of acute Chagas' disease cases are mild.[7] However, in a few percent of cases, an acutely infected person (mostly infants, small children, and immunocompromised individuals) may become seriously ill.[8] Complications may affect the heart (myocarditis, congestive heart failure) and nervous system (meningoencephalitis) and may even cause death.[1,8-12] In about one-third of *T. cruzi* infections, a chronic form of disease develops some 10 to 20 years later, causing irreversible damage to the heart, esophagus, and colon, with dilatation and disorders of nerve conduction of these organs. Patients with severe chronic disease become progressively more ill and ultimately die, usually from heart failure. There is, at present, no effective treatment for such cases.[1,5]

Transfusion-Transmitted Chagas' Disease

Transfusion accounts for the second most common mechanism of *T. cruzi* disease spread in Latin America.[2,13-17] Table 7-2

Table 7-2. Estimates of Blood Donations, Seroprevalence, Screening Coverage, and Number of Potential Cases for *T. cruzi* in Latin America in 1997[18]

Country	Number of Blood Donations	Seroprevalence in Blood Donors (%)	Screening Coverage (%)	Potential Cases
Chile	220,686	79.8	79.8	16
Columbia	422,300	11.1	99.9	2
Costa Rica	58,436	25.7	6.9	487
Ecuador	110,619	1.3	72.3	9
El Salvador	34,091	19.0	100.0	0
Honduras	27,963	11.9	99.0	1
Nicaragua	46,539	3.9	62.1	21
Panama	42,342	NA	NA	NA
Paraguay	39,904	37.7	100.0	0
Peru	203,690	2.0	60.0	36
Uruguay	115,490	6.5	100.0	0
Venezuela	262,295	7.8	100.0	0

gives estimates of blood donations, seroprevalence, screening coverage, and number of potential cases for *T. cruzi* in Latin America in 1997.

In contrast to the situation in Latin America, in the US, transfusion is the most common mechanism of *T. cruzi* disease spread. Although it is true that *T.* cruzi-infected reduviid bugs are found in certain regions of the US, only a handful of cases of Chagas' disease have been attributed to direct vector contact.[19,20] The occurrence of transfusion-transmitted *T. cruzi* in the US is the result of blood donation by *T. cruzi*-infected individuals who qualify as blood donors, in spite of being parasitemic.[1,21] Currently there are approximately 50,000 to

100,000 *T.* cruzi-infected persons in the US,[22-24] and their distribution within the US is not uniform. In some areas, nearly one in every 300 Latin American immigrants who meet Food and Drug Administration (FDA) and AABB donor eligibility criteria may be infected with *T. cruzi.*[25-27] Transmission of Chagas' disease by transfusion has been gaining attention in the US due to at least six transfusion-transmitted cases of acute Chagas' disease in the US and Canada (see Table 7-3).[9-12,28-31]

One has to wonder why more cases of transfusion-transmitted *T. cruzi* have not been reported, given the relatively high frequency of potentially infected blood components, especially in areas such as Los Angeles and Miami, where more than 1 in every 9000 blood donations are from individuals who are seropositive for *T. cruzi*, and polymerase chain reaction (PCR) studies indicate that at least half of *T. cruzi* seropositive donations may contain parasites.[32] The most likely answer to this question is that the symptoms of the acute infection are usually mild and nonspecific, causing US physicians (who do not consider Chagas' disease high on their differential list) to miss and under-report the diagnosis.

Factors that influence the risk of transfusion-transmitted Chagas' disease in the US include the following: 1) para-

Table 7-3. Transfusion-Transmitted Chagas' Disease Diagnosed in the United States and Canada

Year	Location of Case	Origin of Donor
1987	California	Mexico
1989	New York City	Bolivia
1989	Manitoba	Paraguay
1993	Houston	Unknown
1999	Miami	Chile
2000	Manitoba	Germany/Paraguay

sitemia at the time of blood donation, 2) virulence of the parasite, 3) kind and volume of blood component administered, and 4) immunologic status of the recipient.[1] In five of the six cases of transfusion-transmitted Chagas' disease reported to date in the US and Canada, platelet units were implicated as the source of the recipients' *T. cruzi* infections.[1,9,10,12,30] In the other case, the implicated donor could not be determined.[11,33] Therefore, platelets appear to be the most likely blood component to transmit *T. cruzi* infection in the US.[33,34] In Southern California, about 1 in every 93,000 plateletpheresis donations is reportedly positive for *T. cruzi* antibodies, compared with a greater than 10-fold higher incidence in whole blood donations (from which standard platelet concentrates might be made).[31] Thus, it is possible that platelet concentrates produced from whole blood donations present a greater risk of transmitting *T. cruzi* than do plateletpheresis units. Even if an infected unit is transfused, it does not guarantee that the recipient will become infected. For example, it has been estimated that the likelihood of transmitting infection following the transfusion of a *T. cruzi* seropositive blood component is only 20% in Latin America.[13] The experience seen to date in the US using information from look-back investigations suggests an even lower level of infectivity.[29,35]

In addition to vector and transfusion transmission, there may also be congenital infections,[35] infections following solid organ transplantation[36,37] (including three patients in the US who received organs from a single donor),[38] and infections following marrow transplantation.[39,40] There is also a concern regarding Chagas' disease potentially complicating hematopoietic progenitor cell therapy.[41]

Strategies to Prevent Transfusion-Transmitted Chagas' Disease

The fundamental risk factor for transfusion-transmitted Chagas' disease in the US is the collection of donated blood from infected individuals. The distribution of *T. cruzi* seropositive blood donors varies within the US from none to nearly 150 per 100,000 donors.[20,22,25,27,29,34,35,42,43] In some major metropolitan areas, seropositive rates are 1 in 7500 (Los Angeles) and 1 in 9000 (Miami),[22,29] with hot spots of seropositivity in communities such as East Los Angeles where more than 1 of every 1000 eligible blood donors may be seropositive for specific antibodies to *T. cruzi.*[25,27,42] Strategies to prevent transfusion-transmitted *T. cruzi* need to take into account this uneven distribution of risk; however, it is important to realize that even though the likelihood of collecting blood from a *T. cruzi*-infected donor may be regionally dependent, blood components are shipped between geographic regions of the US, so that a unit infected with *T. cruzi* could be distributed to an area where the collection of infected blood would be unlikely.

Donor History Screening Questions

In the US, the current policy is to ask prospective blood donors about a history of Chagas' disease, which is cause for deferral. Asking additional questions upon which to base donor deferral decisions (such as place of birth, travel history, living conditions, or receipt of transfusions while in an area where the disease is endemic) is not generally done. However, the application of a questionnaire to explore the above additional questions has been shown to be effective in detecting (and interdicting) *T. cruzi* seropositive (and presumably parasitemic) blood donors.[27,29,42]

It is possible that some of the reported cases of transfusion-transmitted Chagas' disease might have been prevented if more comprehensive donor screening questions had been employed. There is not consensus on this point, and collegial discussions regarding the use of more extensive questions to interdict *T. cruzi*-infected donors has been debated on the internet at the following URLs: http://www.cbbsweb.org/

enetchagasDonors.html and http://www.cbbsweb.org/enetchagas.html (as of June, 2003).

Although predonation questions identify persons at high risk for infection, donor questioning is probably not sensitive enough to prevent all transfusion-transmitted Chagas' disease, nor specific enough to avoid deferral of excessive numbers of healthy individuals. Studies performed by the American Red Cross with blood donors in Miami and Los Angeles demonstrate that a percentage of *T. cruzi* seropositive donations do slip through a predonation screening process.[29] In the American Red Cross studies, donors were stratified according to risk for *T. cruzi* infection on the basis of answers to questions about history of birth or extended stay in countries where Chagas' disease is endemic. A total of 299,398 donors were queried, and 23,978 reported having a risk factor. The remaining 275,420 donors reported no risk factor. The 23,978 "at-risk" donors and 25,587 of the "no-risk" donors were tested for *T. cruzi* seropositivity. *T. cruzi* specific antibodies were confirmed in 34 donors (in 33 of the "at-risk" donors and in one of the "no-risk" donors) for an overall seroprevalence of about 1 per 9000 donors.[29] Retrospectively, it was found that the seropositive "no-risk" donor had failed to disclose risk factors that would have placed this donor in the "at-risk" group. Seropositivity was 35 times more likely in the "at-risk" donor group (1 in every 727 donors) than in the "no-risk" group (1 in every 25,587 donors).

If the seropositivity rate for "no-risk" donors were to be extrapolated over the entire group of 275,420 "no-risk" donors, it would follow that 11 of the 275,420 "no-risk" donors might be seropositive. Based on this extrapolation, the 33 seropositive "at-risk" donors would represent only 75% of an estimated 44 potentially infected donors (33 seropositive "at-risk" donors + 1 seropositive "no-risk" donor + 10 additional seropositive "no-risk" donors based on an extrapolation). Thus, a donor screen for *T. cruzi* risk factors might defer only 75% of *T. cruzi* seropositive (and presumably parasitemic) donors from donating blood, yet result in the deferral of up to 8% of healthy donors in the Los Angeles and Miami areas, which could negatively affect blood availability.

In another study, Leiby and colleagues identified three *T. cruzi* seropositive blood donors in the Waco, Texas area where an estimated rate of confirmed seropositivity is 1 in 7700.[35] Two of these three donors reported having no risk factors for *T. cruzi* infection, both having been born in the US and neither having traveled to an area where Chagas' disease is endemic. Both donors had extensive family histories of cardiac disease. Therefore, the authors speculated that these two seropositive donors acquired their infections congenitally. The above data and experience support serologic testing, in addition to the use of more extensive questions, in areas of the US where there are large numbers of people who have lived where Chagas' disease is endemic.

Several cases of transfusion-transmitted *T. cruzi* and seroprevalence data suggest a risk as high as 1:7500 of collecting a donor unit from an infected individual in some large cities. However, a policy to test donors for evidence of *T. cruzi* infection is not currently employed in the US because no serologic test for screening blood donors has been approved by the FDA.[44] According to a report from the Blood Products Advisory Committee Meeting of September 12, 2002, where the regulatory pathway and standards for approval of a blood donor screening Chagas' test were discussed, the FDA has not recommended serologic screening for Chagas' disease because of the perceptions that the prevalence of antibody in the donor population is low and that current prevention measures are being achieved by the standard donor questionnaire.[45] Furthermore, there exists no suitably sensitive and specific blood donor screening test. Although FDA-approved enzyme immunoassay (EIA) kits using *T. cruzi* epimastigote (insect form of the parasite) lysate are available for the diagnosis of Chagas' disease in patients with confirmatory testing performed using a radioimmunoprecipitation assay (RIPA), none of these tests are licensed for screening blood donors.

Characteristics of a Blood Donor Screening Test for Chagas's Disease

In the same summary report from the above-cited Blood Products Advisory Committee meeting,[45] the following information was purported to be the current thinking regarding standards for approval of a blood donor screening Chagas' test, assuming the test will be an antigen-based, antibody detection assay similar to the diagnostic tests.

Chemistry, Manufacturing, and Control

In the case of parasite crude lysates, an adequate device should have manufacturing controls that would ensure lot-to-lot consistency of antigen composition. Controls should include use of, but are not limited to, a standard reference panel of sera with varying degrees of reactivity for comparison and quality control of each lot. Western blot testing with these sera should show consistent representation of the immunodominant antigens. Endpoint titration curves from testing of the final product using a panel of sera that exhibit reactivity with the immunodominant antigens should have slopes and midpoints that fall within validated acceptable limits. The *Draft Points to Consider in the Manufacture and Clinical Evaluation of In Vitro Tests to Detect Antibodies to the Human Immunodeficiency Virus Type 1*[46] is a guide to the general quality control procedures. In the case of well-characterized recombinant antigens or peptides, to ensure lot-to-lot consistency, characterization of the product by way of amino acid analysis and peptide sequence should be established. Acceptance criteria and specifications should be established for either type of antigen lots.

Clinical Sensitivity

First, a substantial number (at least 100) of serum samples from patients who are diagnosed parasitologically positive should be tested under an investigational new drug (IND) protocol. The sera are presumed positive; therefore, all sera testing negative by the IND test should be retested by a confirmatory test (RIPA). Second, a prospective study should be performed on a larger number (at least 500) of samples from an area where *T. cruzi* prevalence is > 5%. The prospective study should include a reference test [such as an immunofluorescence assay (IFA)] on each sample. Samples positive on either the IND or reference test should be subjected to a confirmatory test (RIPA).

Clinical Specificity

The assay should be tested in the end user setting with the US population. The assay should be tested at three geographically separated sites, with a large enough number of samples for statistical power (5000 have been sufficient in other studies) at each site using at least three lots of the assay. No reference test is needed; donors are presumed negative. All reactive samples should be confirmed (RIPA).

Analytical Specificity

Preclinical testing should be performed with potential cross-reactive sera such as that from patients infected with *Leishmania*. Potential interfering serum samples should be spiked with positive sera such that the final dilution of the Chagas' antibody is near the cut-off. Test results with such spiked sera should be compared to tests of positive samples without potential interfering sera for sensitivity and specificity.

Analytical Sensitivity

Tests should be performed on dilution series of positive samples and seroconversion panels, if available.

Reproducibility/Proficiency

A panel of at least five sera composed of positive, negative, and weakly reactive sera should be tested in at least three sites with different operators with at least three lots of the assay.

Instrument/Software

Instruments and software are medical devices that should be developed and manufactured in accordance with the Quality System regulation (21 CFR 820). The FDA Center for Devices and Radiological Health (CDRH) guidance document *General Principles of Software Validation*[47] may be used to assist with software-related design control issues. The instrument and software portion of the application require a separate 510(k) submission. The CDRH *Guidance for the Content of Premarket Submissions for Software Contained in Medical Devices*[48] contains all of the submission requirements for software applications. This type of device would be considered a major level of concern because the assay will be a licensed test used for screening blood donors.

Testing Options

Testing a Subset of Donors

If and when a Chagas' disease screening test approved by the FDA becomes available for blood donor testing, some centers might wish to test only a subset of selected donors. If such a policy were followed, only a limited number of individuals would need to be tested, which would minimize cost, the occurrence of false-negative EIA results, and the deferral of otherwise healthy individuals. This type of policy seems reasonable based on data from Los Angeles and Miami, where donors who reported risk factors for *T. cruzi* infection were about 35 times more likely to test positive for *T. cruzi* antibodies than donors who reported no risk. There is precedent for selective testing of a subset of donated blood. For example, not all donors are tested for evidence of antibodies to cytomegalovirus (CMV). However, the testing of donors for CMV antibodies is based on the characteristics of the transfusion recipient, not on the presence or absence of donor risk factors.

The size and composition of the subset of donors tested would depend on the demographics of the donor group and on which screening question(s) were used. For example, if only those donors who had a risk factor for classic *T. cruzi* infection were selected for testing (ie, the donor reported having Chagas' disease, living in close contact with infected insects, and/or receiving a transfusion in a country where Chagas' disease is endemic), the subgroup needing testing would be very small. A report[49] from California showed that the median prevalence of at least one risk factor for classic *T. cruzi* infection among blood donors was 0.33%, based on a survey of 17,521 blood donors from 18 California blood collection centers. Fifty-seven of the donors (1 of every 307 donors) had one or more risk factors for *T. cruzi* infection; 39 donors had lived in dwellings with mud walls or thatched roofs; 16 donors had received transfusions in areas where Chagas' disease was endemic; and six donors had been diagnosed with Chagas' disease. Donors at risk for *T. cruzi* were found in all 18 collection centers studied. According to data from the LAC+USC Medical Center Blood Bank (one of the participating centers in Galel's study), prospective donors with one or more risk factors for classic *T. cruzi* infection had a 3% to 4% likelihood of being seropositive for specific antibodies to *T. cruzi*. Thus, the testing of such a highly selective subgroup of individuals would be expected to detect seropositive donors at a rate of 1 per 25 to 1 per 33 "high-risk" donors tested. The problem with such an approach is that it requires the use of a special set of questions, which adds complexity and time to the predonation screening process.[27,42]

If a policy was implemented to test a subset of donors based on less specific criteria, such as birth or extended stay in a Chagas'-disease-endemic area for more than 1 year, then the subgroup tested would be larger, but the process of questioning donors for risk factors would be simplified. With this approach, about 2.4% of California blood donors would require testing. Because at-risk individuals tend to be concentrated in metropolitan areas, about 8% of donors in Los Angeles and Miami would fall into a subgroup needing testing. Close to 40% of donors from East Los Angeles would require testing.[42]

Limiting Repeat Testing for Seronegative Donors

Another variation on the theme of selective testing would be to test each donor's *T. cruzi* serostatus once, regardless of risk factors. A donor who was shown to be *T. cruzi* seronegative would not need to be retested for *T. cruzi* antibodies, unless the donor subsequently received a blood transfusion and/or traveled to a country where Chagas' disease is endemic. If a seronegative donor received a transfusion or traveled to such a country, after an appropriate temporary deferral period (such as 1 year), the donor could be retested for *T. cruzi* antibodies at a subsequent donation to ensure a *T. cruzi* infection had not been acquired. A 1-year deferral would have a minimal impact on the blood supply because most countries in Latin America where Chagas' disease is endemic are also where malaria is endemic. Following a blood transfusion, donors are already deferred for 1 year. A year's deferral allows adequate time for antibody development, in the event the donor became infected with *T. cruzi*. There are data to suggest that seroconversion to *T. cruzi* is detectable within a year following infection.[30] For example, following the accidental release and shipment of a *T. cruzi* seropositive unit of platelets, the blood component was transfused to a 60-year-old multiple myeloma patient. The transfusion recipient became infected as demonstrated by the development of an antibody response and by the finding of parasitemia demonstrated by PCR and hemoculture. Serum samples from the patient before transfusion and at day 43 after transfusion were negative for antibodies to *T. cruzi* by EIA. At day 57 after transfusion, the recipient was EIA seronegative, but positive by hemoculture and by PCR. Subsequent samples at day 95, 100, and 127 after transfusion were all PCR and hemoculture positive. The day 95 serum sample was just below the EIA cutoff, but a day 100 sample was repeatedly reactive; both samples were negative in confirmatory testing. The serum sample from day 127 was unsuitable for testing. The patient was reported to have *no clinical signs* of disease and was not treated for acute Chagas' disease.

The patient eventually died, but the death was stated to be unrelated to *T. cruzi* infection. The blood donor was born in Chile and had emigrated to the US 33 years before the blood donation in question. The platelet donor was also parasitemic, as demonstrated by PCR.

Testing All Donations

A policy to test each blood donor for *T. cruzi* antibodies at every blood donation would probably be the least complicated operational approach and would be the most standardized of the various testing schemes. If a *T. cruzi* antibody test were licensed for donor screening, FDA regulations might prohibit a selective testing approach. The agency might view the selective testing of donor subgroups to be contrary to good manufacturing practice principles. The universal testing of donors for *T. cruzi* antibodies would, however, result in the greatest number of false-positive tests and the greatest expense for testing. Unless the occurrence of clerical errors increased because an additional test was added to the donor testing routine, a universal testing approach should detect the greatest number of seropositive donors and minimize the transfusion of seropositive blood components.

Nontesting Approaches

Leukocyte Reduction

Until a *T. cruzi* antibody test for screening blood donors is available, one might consider using leukocyte-reduced blood components exclusively. A study by Moraes-Souza and colleagues[50] investigated the efficacy of leukocyte reduction filters in removing *T. cruzi* from infected blood. Human blood was contaminated with 2 or 150 *T. cruzi* parasites per mL and then left unfiltered or filtered with leukocyte reduction filters that provided either 2, 3, or 6 log removal of leukocytes. The efficacy of the parasite removal of these filters was evaluated by microscopic enumeration of active forms of *T. cruzi* both in vivo and in vitro. The in-vivo experiments were performed with Swiss mice that had been intraperitoneally inoculated with *T. cruzi*-infected human blood. The in-vitro experiments were performed with fresh human blood that had been deliberately contaminated with *T. cruzi*. The number of parasites seen in mice inoculated with the unfiltered blood was significantly higher than the number of parasites seen in mice inoculated with blood from the same sample that had been filtered to cause a 3 or 6 log removal of leukocytes. Fifty to 70 percent of the mice given *T. cruzi*-infected (2 parasites/mL) filtered blood did not develop *T. cruzi* infection. In vitro, the use of leukocyte reduction filters, providing 2, 3, or 6 log leukocyte removal, significantly reduced the number of parasites seen in culture.

The present experimental data suggest that leukocyte reduction filters are effective in reducing the number of parasites in *T. cruzi*-infected blood. This efficacy depends, in part, on the concentration of parasites in the artificially infected blood. These data do not address whether leukocyte reduction by a nonfiltration method would be effective in reducing the number of *T. cruzi* parasites in platelets. This is an important question because the preferred method for leukocyte reduction of plateletpheresis units is by differential centrifugation, and not by leukocyte filtration. Studies will need to be performed to determine if leukocyte-reduced plateletpheresis units prepared without leukocyte reduction filters have a comparable reduction in risk compared with platelets that are leukocyte reduced using these filters. Clinical studies will also need to be performed to determine if the risk of transfusion-transmitted Chagas' disease is reduced by the routine use of leukocyte-reduced blood components (regardless of the method of leukocyte reduction).

Chemical Treatment

Another nontesting approach to prevent transfusion-transmitted Chagas' disease might be to add a chemical, such as gentian violet, to the blood component to kill the parasite.

Gentian violet has been shown to be effective and is currently the only in-vitro trypanocidal agent. The use of gentian violet in the chemoprophylaxis of transfusion-transmitted Chagas' disease is strongly recommended in areas where Chagas' disease is endemic, but where serologic tests are not available.[51] Unfortunately, gentian violet causes the plasma in the blood component to change its color, which can cause a transient discoloration of the skin of the recipient. Also, the long-term toxicity of this agent for blood recipients remains an open issue.[52]

A colorless, nontoxic, and efficient drug to prevent transfusion-associated Chagas' disease may have recently been described in the form of an aminoquinolone named "WR6026."[53] Investigators of this drug's effects on the metabolism of red cells stored with this compound suggest that WR6026 does not interfere in the preservation and probably the viability of the erythrocytes until day 28 of storage; the authors suggest that WR6026 could emerge as a colorless substitute for gentian violet in the control of transfusion-associated Chagas' disease in endemic areas of Latin America.[53] It is unlikely, however, that the FDA would approve either gentian violet or WR6026 to prevent transfusion-transmitted Chagas' disease. The magnitude of this problem may not justify such a drastic approach, and serologic testing or leukocyte reduction strategies may reduce the risk to essentially zero without chemical treatment of blood components.

Summary and Recommendations

Current data are insufficient to define the true risk of transfusion-transmitted Chagas' disease in the US. Experience suggests that the virulence of the *T. cruzi* strain(s) present in donated blood and/or the level of parasitemia among infected blood donors in the US may be too low to establish infection in most (but not all) recipients. However, because it is well documented that transfusion-transmitted Chagas' disease has occurred on multiple occasions in the US and Canada, it would seem prudent to implement a policy to prevent the transfusion of additional *T. cruzi*-infected blood components. A policy to elicit risk factors (such as living conditions or transfusion history in Latin America) would likely detect nearly 75% of the highest risk individuals. However, such questioning alone will not detect all infected individuals because some prospective donors acquired their infection in the US via vector contact, transfusion, or even congenitally. In addition, some donors do not report their risk factors, even when asked about them during donor screening. Thus, testing blood donors for *T. cruzi* antibodies would be a more effective intervention strategy than questioning donors for *T. cruzi* risk factors. Testing donors for evidence of *T. cruzi* infection would probably be effective if each donor was tested to establish his or her serologic baseline status. Once found to be negative, donors would not need to be retested unless they traveled to an area where Chagas' disease is endemic or they received a blood transfusion. Alternatively, if it was too difficult to keep track of a donor's baseline serologic status, testing could be performed on each donation. In the event that the FDA does not license a screening test for *T. cruzi*, the routine use of leukocyte-reduced blood components might be sufficient, if it was proven that the use of leukocyte-reduced blood components lowered the risk of transfusion-transmitted *T. cruzi* infection to nearly zero.

References

1. Gudino MD, Linares J. Chagas' disease and blood transfusion. In: Westphal RG, Carlson KB, Turc JM, eds. Emerging global patterns in transfusion-transmitted infections. Arlington, VA: American Association of Blood Banks, 1990:65-85.
2. Schmunis GA. *Trypanosoma cruzi*, the etiologic agent of Chagas' disease: Status in the blood supply in endemic and nonendemic countries. Transfusion 1991;31:547-57.
3. Kirchhoff LV. *Trypanosoma* species (American trypanosomiasis, Chagas disease): Biology of trypanosomes. In: Mandell GL, Bennett JE, eds. Principles and practice of infectious diseases. 4th ed. New York: Churchill Livingstone, 1995:2442-50.
4. Control of Chagas disease: Report of a WHO expert committee. WHO Tech Rep Ser 1991;811:27-37.

5. Centers for Disease Control and Prevention. Annex A. Fact sheets for candidate diseases for elimination or eradication. MMWR Morb Mortal Wkly Rep 1999;48(SU01):154-203.
6. Chagas—recent epidemiological data. [Available at http://www.who. int/ctd/chagas/epidemio.htm.]
7. Kirchhoff LV. Chagas disease. American trypanosomiasis. Infect Dis Clin North Am 1993;7(3):487-502.
8. Kirchhoff LV. American trypanosomiasis (Chagas' disease)—a tropical disease now in the United States. N Engl J Med 1993;329:639-44.
9. Geiseler PJ, Ito JI, Tegtmeier BR, et al. Fulminant Chagas disease (CD) in bone marrow transplantation (BMT) (abstract). In: Abstracts of the 27th Interscience Conference on Antimicrobial Agents and Chemotherapy. Washington, DC: American Society for Microbiology, 1987: 169.
10. Grant IH, Gold JWM, Wittner M, et al. Transfusion-associated acute Chagas disease acquired in the United States. Ann Intern Med 1989; 111:849-51.
11. Cimo PL, Luper WE, Scouros MA. Transfusion-associated Chagas' disease in Texas: Report of a case. Texas Med 1993;89:48-50.
12. Nickerson P, Orr P, Schroeder M, et al. Transfusion-associated *Trypanosoma cruzi* infection in a non-endemic area. Ann Intern Med 1989;111:851-3.
13. Schmunis GA. Prevention of transfusional *Trypanosoma cruzi* infection in Latin America. Mem Inst Oswaldo Cruz 1999;94(Suppl 1):93-101.
14. Saez-Alquezar A, Otani MM, Sabino EC, et al. Evaluation of the performance of Brazilian blood banks in testing for Chagas' disease. Vox Sang 1998;74:228-31.
15. Salles NA, Sabino EC, Cliquet MG, et al. Risk of exposure to Chagas' disease among seroreactive Brazilian blood donors. Transfusion 1996; 36:969-73.
16. Schmunis GA, Zicker F, Pinheiro F, Brandling-Bennett D. Risk for transfusion-transmitted infectious diseases in Central and South America. Emerg Infect Dis 1998;4:5-11.
17. Umezawa ES, Corbett CE, Shikanai-Yasuda MA, Stolf AM. Chagas' disease. Lancet 2001;357:797-9.
18. Goodnough LT, Shander A, Brecher ME. Transfusion medicine: Looking to the future. Lancet 2003;361:161-9.
19. Ochs DE, Hnilica V, Moser DR, et al. Postmortem PCR-based diagnosis of autochthonous acute Chagas myocarditis in the United States. Am J Trop Med Hyg 1996;34:526-9.
20. Barrett VJ, Leiby DA, Odom JL, et al. Negligible prevalence of antibodies against Trypanosoma cruzi among blood donors in the southeastern United States. Am J Clin Pathol 1997;108:499-503.
21. Wendel S. Current concepts on transmission of bacteria and parasites by blood components. Vox Sang 1994;67(Suppl 3):161-74.
22. Leiby DA, Herron RM, Read EJ, et al. *Trypanosoma cruzi* in Los Angeles and Miami blood donors: Impact of evolving donor demographics on

seroprevalence and implications for transfusion transmission. Transfusion 2002;42:549-55.

23. Kirchhoff LV, Gam AA, Gilliam FC. American trypanosomiasis (Chagas' disease) in Central American immigrants. Am J Med 1987;82 (5):915-20.
24. Schmunis GA. *Trypanosoma cruzi,* the etiological agent of Chagas' disease as a contaminant of blood supplies. A problem of endemic and nonendemic countries. Transfusion 1991;31:547-57.
25. Kerndt P, Waskin HA, Kirchhoff LV, et al. Prevalence of antibody to *Trypanosoma cruzi* among blood donors in Los Angeles, California. Transfusion 1991;31:814-18.
26. Pan AA, Brashear RJ, Schur JD, et al. Chagas' disease among blood donors in North and South America. The prevalence of seroreactive antibodies to *Trypanosoma cruzi* in the United States and Argentina (abstract). Transfusion 1992;32(Suppl):65S.
27. Appleman MD, Shulman IA, Saxena S, Kirchhoff LV. Use of a questionnaire to identify potential blood donors at risk for infection with *Trypanosoma cruzi*. Transfusion 1993;33:61-4.
28. Leiby DA, Lenes BA, Tibbals MA, et al. Prospective evaluation of a patient with *Trypanosoma cruzi* infection transmitted by transfusion. N Engl J Med 1999;341(16):1237-9.
29. Leiby DA, Read EJ, Lenes BA, et al. Seroepidemiology of *Trypanosoma cruzi,* etiologic agent of Chagas' disease, in US blood donors. J Infect Dis 1997;176:1047-52.
30. Lenes BA, Leiby DA, Tibbals MA, Olmedo M. A prospectively identified case of transfusion transmitted *Trypanosoma cruzi*: A defining window period? (abstract) Transfusion 1998;38(Suppl):103S.
31. Leiby DA. Chagas disease. Will Chagas be the next mandated test for screening. Ortho S.E.E.D. Program. August 28, 2002.
32. Tibbals MA, Leiby DA, Herwaldt BL, Herron Jr RM. Evidence of circulating parasites in *Trypanosoma cruzi* seropositive blood donors (abstract).Transfusion 1998;38(Suppl):103S.
33. Shulman IA. Intervention strategies to reduce the risk of transfusion-transmitted *Trypanosoma cruzi* infection in the United States. Transfus Med Rev 1999;13(3):227-34.
34. Leiby DA. Transfusion-transmitted diseases (bacteria and parasites). Latest trends in transfusion-transmitted parasitic infections. In: The Annual Meeting Compendium. Bethesda, MD: American Association of Blood Banks, 1998:332-6.
35. Leiby DA, Fucci MH, Stumpf RJ. *Trypanosoma cruzi* in a low to moderate risk blood donor population: Seroprevalence and possible congenital transmission. Transfusion 1999;39(3):310-15.
36. Ferraz AS, Figueiredo JF. Transmission of Chagas' disease through transplanted kidney: Occurrence of the acute form of the disease in two recipients from the same donor. Rev Inst Med Trop Sao Paulo 1993;35(5):461-3.

37. Carvalho MF, de Franco MF, Soares VA. Amastigote forms of *Trypanosoma cruzi* detected in a renal allograft. Rev Inst Med Trop Sao Paulo 1997;39(4):223-6.
38. Zayas CF, Perlino C, Caliendo A, et al. Chagas' disease after organ transplantation—United States 2001. MMWR Morb Mortal Wkly Rep 2002;51(10):210-2.
39. Altclas J, Jaimovich G, Milovic V, et al. Chagas' disease after bone marrow transplantation. Bone Marrow Transplant 1996;18(2):447-8.
40. Villalba R, Fornes G, Alvarez MA, et al. Acute Chagas' disease in a recipient of a bone marrow transplant in Spain: Case report. Clin Infect Dis 1992 Feb;14(2):594-5.
41. Centers for Disease Control and Prevention. Guidelines for preventing opportunistic infections among hematopoietic stem cell transplant recipients. Recommendations of Centers for Disease Control and Prevention, the Infectious Disease Society of America, and the American Society of Blood and Marrow Transplantation. MMWR Morb Mortal Wkly Rep 2000;49(RR10);1-128.
42. Shulman IA, Appleman MD, Saxena S, et al. Specific antibodies to *Trypanosoma cruzi* among blood donors in Los Angeles, California. Transfusion 1997;37(7):727-31.
43. Brashear RJ, Winkler MA, Schur JD, et al. Detection of antibodies to Trypanosoma cruzi among blood donors in the southwestern and western United States. I. Evaluation of the sensitivity and specificity of an enzyme immunoassay for detecting antibodies to *T. cruzi*. Transfusion 1995;35(3):213-18.
44. Leiby DA, Wendel S, Takaoka DT, et al. Serologic testing for *Trypanosoma cruzi*: Comparison of radioimmunoprecipitation assay with commercially available indirect immunofluorescence assay, indirect hemagglutination assay, and enzyme-linked immunosorbent assay kits. J Clin Microbiol 2000;38(2):639-42.
45. Duncan R. Current trends in transfusion-transmitted Chagas' disease in USA and the regulatory pathway for the approval of Chagas testing for blood donor screening. Presented at FDA Blood Products Advisory Committee meeting, September 21, 2002. [Available at http://www. fda.gov/ohrms/dockets/ac/02/briefing/3892b1.htm].
46. Food and Drug Administration. Draft points to consider in the manufacture and clinical evaluation of in vitro tests to detect antibodies to the human immunodeficiency virus, type 1 (August 8, 1989). Rockville, MD: CBER Office of Communication, Training, and Manufacturers Assistance, 1989. [Available at http://www.fda.gov/cber/gdlns/ptc-hiv1.pdf.]
47. Food and Drug Administration. General principles of software validation: Final guidance for industry and FDA staff. Rockville, MD: CBER Office of Communication, Training, and Manufacturers Assistance, 2002. [Available at http://www.fda.gov/cdrh/comp/guidance/938.html.]

48. Food and Drug Administration. Guidance for the content of premarket submissions for software contained in medical devices. (May 29, 1998) Rockville, MD: CDRH Division of Small Manufacturers, International, and Consumer Assistance, 1998. [Available at http://www.fda.gov/cdrh/ode/57.html.]
49. Galel S, Kirchhoff LV. Risk factors for *Trypanosoma cruzi* infection in California blood donors. Transfusion 1996;36:227-31.
50. Moraes-Souza H, Bordin JO, Bardossy L, et al. Prevention of transfusion-associated Chagas disease: Efficacy of white cell-reduction filters in removing *Trypanosoma cruzi* from infected blood. Transfusion 1995; 35(9):723-6.
51. Moraes-Souza H, Kerbauy J, Barretto OC, et al. Metabolism and preservation of fresh and stored erythrocytes in blood treated with gentian violet. Braz J Med Biol Res 1988;21(2):241-6.
52. Moraes-Souza H, Bordin JO. Strategies for prevention of transfusion-associated Chagas' disease. Transfus Med Rev 1996;10:161-70.
53. Moraes-Souza H, Pianetti GM, Barretto OC, et al. Aminoquinolone WR6026 as a feasible substitute for gentian violet in Chagas' disease prophylaxis in preserved blood for transfusional purposes. Rev Soc Bras Med Trop 2002;35(6):563-9.

In: Brecher ME, ed.
Bacterial and Parasitic Contamination of Blood Components
Bethesda, MD: AABB Press, 2003

8

Babesia and Other Parasites

DAVID A. LEIBY, PHD

FOR MANY YEARS, DISCUSSIONS OF PARASITIC agents and the safety of the blood supply have focused on *Plasmodium* spp. and *Trypanosoma cruzi*, the etiologic agents of malaria and Chagas' disease, respectively. These parasitic agents, first recognized approximately 100 years ago, have been closely monitored and evaluated over the last several decades to better understand the threats they pose to blood safety. Thus, it is fitting that this book reviews blood contamination by *Plasmodium* spp. and *T.*

David A. Leiby, PhD, Chief of Parasitology, Transmissible Diseases Department, Jerome H. Holland Laboratory for the Biomedical Sciences, American Red Cross, Rockville, Maryland, and Associate Professor of Microbiology and Tropical Medicine, George Washington University, Washington, District of Columbia cruzi in separate, in-depth chapters. However, there are several other parasitic agents that affect blood safety with increasing regularity.

Indeed, there are a number of parasitic agents that have only recently emerged as threats to blood safety. These emergent agents pose new and unique challenges to the safety of the blood supply; however, only limited surveillance and epidemiologic information is available for these agents. Foremost among these emergent agents are several transmitted by ticks including *Babesia* spp., *Ehrlichia chaffeensis*, and *Anaplasma phagocytophilum*—the agents of human babesiosis, human monocytic ehrlichiosis (HME), and human granulocytic ehrlichiosis (HGE), respectively (Table 8-1). This chapter focuses on these three tick-borne agents, reviewing the latest information on their epidemiology, clinical symptoms, diagnosis, treatment, seroprevalence, transfusion transmission, and, as appropriate, measures to control their transmission. Additionally, this chapter briefly discusses other parasitic agents (eg, *Leishmania* spp., *Toxoplasma gondii*, etc) that have been recognized for many years but likely pose a minimal threat to blood safety.

Babesia Spp.

Epidemiology

Members of the genus *Babesia* are intraerythrocytic protozoan parasites that cause the zoonotic disease babesiosis. Human infections attributable to *Babesia* spp. have been reported from the United States, Europe, Latin America, Africa, and Southeast Asia.[1] Despite the parasite's wide distribution, the majority of human cases have been reported in the United States and Europe. The first case of human babesiosis in the United States occurred in 1966.[2] Since then, hundreds of human cases have been reported in the United States, and the numbers continue to increase as the endemic range of the parasite expands.

Nearly all US cases of human babesiosis can be attributed to infections with the rodent babesial parasite, *B. microti*.[3,4] In the

Table 8-1. Characteristics of the Primary Tick-Borne Parasitic Agents That Pose Blood Safety Risks

Disease/Agent	Primary Area of Endemicity	Vector	Transfusion Cases
Babesiosis			
Babesia microti	US (Northeast, Upper Midwest)	*Ixodes scapularis*	>50
WA-1	US (Pacific Coast)	*I. pacificus* (?)	2
Babesia divergens	Europe	*I. ricinus*	NR
Human monocytic ehrlichiosis			
Ehrlichia chaffeensis	US	*Amblyomma americanun*	NR
Human granulocytic ehrlichiosis			
Anaplasma phagocytophilum	US	*I. scapularis, I. pacificus*	1
	Europe	*I. ricinus*	NR

NR = none reported.

United States, *B. microti* is endemic to the Upper Midwest and Northeast, with human cases reported as far south as New Jersey.[5] During the last 10 years, human cases attributable to emerging *Babesia*-like organisms have been reported in Washington, California, and Missouri; these agents have been designated as WA-1, CA-1, and MO-1, respectively.[6-8] More recently, the first case of human babesiosis caused by the bovine parasite *B. divergens* was reported in the United States.[9] In Europe, *B. divergens* causes most cases of human babesiosis,[10] but *B. bovis*, *B. canis*, and *B. microti* have been implicated in other sporadic human cases.[11]

Human infections with *Babesia* are acquired almost exclusively by contact with an infected tick vector of the *Ixodes* group. In the United States, *B. microti* is transmitted to humans by the black-legged tick, *I. scapularis*, also referred to as the deer tick. Both nymphal and adult stages of the tick are capable of transmitting the parasite during the course of a blood meal. In addition to the tick vector, the white-footed mouse (*Peromyscus leucopus*) and white-tailed deer play pivotal roles in the enzootic life cycle of *B. microti*. The mouse serves as the reservoir host for the parasite, while deer, a noncompetent host for *B. microti*, are an important maintenance and transport host for adults of *I. scapularis*. The life cycle of WA-1 is thought to be similar and the tick vector is purported to be *I. pacificus*.

European cases of human babesiosis, particularly those attributable to *B. divergens*, are thought to be transmitted by the sheep tick, *I. ricinus*.[11] Additionally, *I. ricinus* has been identified as the vector of *B. divergens* among bovines, and perhaps not surprisingly, the incidence of human babesiosis in Europe appears to be greatest where cattle are most numerous. The Japanese vector for the recently reported cases of a *B. microti*-like agent have not been confirmed but by analogy is thought to be *I. persulcatus*, the main vector of Lyme borreliosis in Japan.[12] The reservoir host for the Japanese isolate is thought to be a field mouse (*Adodemus speciosus*).

Because of the central role ticks play in transmitting these agents, active transmission and subsequent disease appearance are seasonal, occurring primarily from May through September (in the Northern Hemisphere) when ticks are actively feeding. Successful transmission of *B. microti* to humans also requires that an infected tick feeds for 48 hours or longer.[13] Thus, the removal of ticks shortly after attachment and before extended feeding can greatly reduce the transmission of *Babesia* spp.

Clinical Symptoms

Successful transmission of *Babesia* spp. occurs when the infective stage or sporozoite reaches maturity in tick salivary glands and is inoculated into the vertebrate host. Once introduced into the host, the sporozoites enter erythrocytes, transform into merozoites, and undergo limited replication via binary fission. An exoerythrocytic stage has not been identified. In most cases, *Babesia* infections produce subclinical illness, but mild acute illness characterized by fever, headache, and myalgias can occur 1 to 4 weeks after the tick bite. More severe cases of disease, particularly among infants and the immunocompromised (eg, asplenic, elderly), can demonstrate hemolytic anemia, thrombocytopenia, renal failure, and mortality rates that approach 5%.[14] Indeed, in asplenic patients, parasitemias can range as high as 85%.[15] Human infections with WA-1 and *B. divergens* are more virulent than those with *B. microti*, causing fulminant cases of disease with rapid onset.[6,11]

Diagnosis and Treatment

The diagnosis of *Babesia* infections is generally accomplished using one or more of the following techniques: direct detection, serology, or polymerase chain reaction (PCR). In its simplest form, direct detection of babesial infection is accomplished by examining stained peripheral blood smears for infected erythrocytes. However, because most cases of babesiosis are characterized by low levels of parasitemia, direct detection by smear often lacks sufficient sensitivity. Additionally, because erythrocytes infected with *Babesia* spp. and *Plasmodium* spp. demonstrate similar morphologies, a clear distinction between these two parasites must be made. The sensitivity of direct detection can be enhanced by inoculating hamsters with patient blood. Hamsters are susceptible to most species of *Babesia* and patient infections are readily demonstrable in smears of hamster blood several weeks after inoculation.

Serologic detection of babesiosis relies primarily on the indirect immunofluorescent assay (IFA), which is capable of detecting IgM and IgG antibodies to *Babesia* spp.[16] The recent development of a sensitive and specific enzyme immunoassay (EIA) for *B. microti* antibodies may provide a rapid and objective method for efficiently testing large numbers of samples.[17] Regardless of whether an IFA or EIA is used, serologic tests are unlikely to detect early acute phase infections, commonly referred to as "window period" infections. PCR assays have been developed that amplify highly conserved sequences of *B. microti, B. divergens,* and WA-1,[18-20] which can be used to identify window period infections as well as cases of persistent parasitemia.[21] Despite the utility of PCR, its sensitivity is limited by sample size, and a negative result does not exclude the possibility of infection, particularly one in which parasites circulate intermittently in the blood or remain lodged in sequestered locations.

Babesial infections are generally treated with a combination of quinine and clindamycin. Unfortunately, adverse reactions to these drugs are not uncommon and can have a negative impact on the effectiveness of treatment. An alternative drug therapy is atovaquone and azithromycin, a combination that has been shown to be equally efficacious in the absence of complicating adverse reactions.[22] When babesiosis is severe or drug treatment fails, exchange transfusion has been successfully used to rapidly reduce parasitemia levels and reverse the course of disease.[23-25]

Seroprevalence

Relatively few studies have been published on the seroprevalence of *Babesia*. These studies were conducted primarily in the United States and examined rates for human infections with *B. microti* and WA-1. Most US studies were conducted in the Northeast, where the seroprevalence rates for *B. microti* ranged from 1.0% to 6.9%.[3] Several studies have reported on *B. microti* rates in blood donors: 3.7% (n = 779) on Cape Cod, 4.3% (n = 115) on Shelter Island (NY), 0.3% (n = 999) in Wisconsin, and 0.3 to 0.6% (n = 1000, n = 1007) in Connecticut.[26-28] Limited studies of WA-1 reported wide ranges of seroprevalence in California and Washington: 0.9% (n = 115) to 17.8% (n = 219).[6,7,29] In the only published study of WA-1 in blood donors, 25 of 124 (20.8%) Sacramento donors were seropositive. Questions have been raised, however, regarding the specificity of WA-1 tests used in these studies.[10] Thus, until WA-1 tests with improved specificity and sensitivity become available, the prevalence of WA-1 among the general population and blood donors remains enigmatic.

Transfusion Transmission

B. microti is the parasitic agent most frequently transmitted by blood transfusion in the United States. It has been suggested that there have been more than 40 cases of transfusion-transmitted *B. microti*,[30] but this number is likely conservative and may now exceed 50. With the exception of transfusion cases reported in Japan and Canada, all *Babesia* transfusion cases have occurred in the United States.[31,32] Even though WA-1 was first described 10 years ago, there have been two confirmed cases of transfusion-transmission involving this agent.[20,33]

Most cases of transfusion-transmitted *B. microti* have involved an asymptomatic blood donor and an immunocompromised recipient, who was often multitransfused and in several cases asplenic.[25] Infected recipients have ranged in age from less than 4 months to 79 years of age. The reported incubation period for transfusion-transmitted babesiosis is 1 to 9 weeks, with symptoms varying from mild to severe, in some cases leading to death. The blood component generally implicated in *B. microti* transfusion cases is Red Blood Cell (RBC) units; however, at least four cases have been attributed to platelets thought to be contaminated with *Babesia*-infected red cells. A 1991-1992 study in Connecticut calculated the risk of acquiring *B. microti* from an RBC unit as 1 in 601 or 0.17% (95% CI, 0.004%-0.9%) and for platelets as 0 in 371 or 0% (95% CI, 0-0.8%).[34] Using different methodology, a more recent Connecticut study calculated the risk of transfusion-transmitted *B. microti* as 1 in 1800 transfused RBC units.[35]

A key factor contributing to the transmission of *B. microti* by blood transfusion is the parasite's ability to survive and remain viable in stored blood components. An infected RBC unit implicated in one *B. microti* transfusion case was 35 days old,[36] indicating that the parasite can survive and remain viable at 4 C for at least 35 days. In laboratory experiments, *B. microti* survived in blood tubes maintained at 4 C for up to 21 days,[37] but this measurement was limited by less than ideal blood storage conditions. Little is known concerning WA-1 survival in blood components, but the most recent transfusion case suggests that this agent can survive for a minimum of 6 days.[33]

Control Strategies

Despite a growing number of transfusion-related babesiosis cases, strategies to prevent transmission of this parasite have not been implemented. It has been suggested that donor-reported tick bites could be used as a basis for donor deferral.[3] However, a recently published study indicated that in some blood collection areas up to 9% of blood donors would need to be deferred—clearly an unacceptable level.[28] Alternatively, one could test only those donors who report a tick bite. However, in the same study, control donors were just as likely to be infected with *B. microti* as those donors reporting a tick bite. Those donors most likely to report a tick bite demonstrate "tick avoidance" behavior (ie, examine themselves for ticks, remove ticks promptly, etc). Moreover, people infected with tick-borne diseases generally do not recall an associated tick bite.[38-40] Thus, risk-factor questions regarding exposure to ticks do not appear to be sufficiently sensitive.

A closely related approach would be to avoid the collection of blood in areas where *B. microti* is endemic during the peak periods of parasite transmission (eg, May-September). However, reports that some people exhibit a chronic carrier state, during which they would be capable of transmitting the parasite year-round, would negate the effectiveness of this approach. Also, deferring large numbers of healthy donors based on a seasonal deferral would seem to be counterproductive. One must also consider that donors who reside in seasonally affected areas could still donate in other locations. Also, donors who become infected during visits or vacations in affected areas may donate blood in areas where *B. microti* is not endemic when they return home.

Blood screening, although an attractive alternative to risk-factor questions, remains problematic. At present, there are no tests licensed to screen blood donations for *B. microti*. The recent report of an EIA test for *B. microti* suggests that suitable tests may be available in the near future.[17] If, and when, blood is screened for *B. microti*, it is unclear what approach will provide the greatest cost/benefit. In the United States, *Babesia* infections remain primarily regionalized in the Northeast and Upper Midwest; thus, universal screening may not be needed. However, given the expanding range of the parasite, the movement of blood components and donors between areas, and the logistical constraints inherent in testing only a portion of the blood supply, regional testing may not be a viable solution.

Given that most cases of babesiosis are either asymptomatic or mild, another approach would be to provide blood recipients who are at the greatest risk for acquiring serious infection with blood components that have tested negative for *B. microti*. A similar strategy is used effectively to limit the transmission of cytomegalovirus. Another consideration for testing is the need to identify those infected donors in the early acute phase or window period. Based on existing PCR assays for *B. microti*, nucleic acid testing is a feasible strategy to identify early infections not recognized by serologic testing.

Two relatively new technologies, leukocyte reduction and pathogen inactivation, are often presented as potential adjuncts or replacements for existing blood safety measures. Leukocyte reduction appears to provide little or no benefit because *Babesia* spp. are intraerythrocytic parasites that would be unaffected by filtration. In contrast, preliminary studies using a pathogen inactivation photosensitizing compound neutralized *B. divergens* in red cells, but the collateral effects (eg, hemolysis) on noninfected cells were not entirely clear.[41]

Ehrlichia chaffeensis and *Anaplasma phagocytophilum*

Epidemiology

The agents of human ehrlichiosis fall into the broad category of rickettsias, a group that includes those agents that cause scrub typhus (*Orientia tsutsugamuchi*) and Rocky Mountain Spotted Fever (*Rickettsia rickettsia*). Five rickettsial agents (gram-negative intracellular parasites of arthropods) are recognized worldwide to cause human cases of ehrlichiosis: *E. sennetsu*, *E. canis*, *E. ewingii*, *E. chaffeensis*, and *A. phagocytophilum*.[42-49] *E. chaffeensis* and *A. phagocytophilum* cause the majority of human ehrlichial infections and at present are the only ehrlichial agents of concern for blood safety.

E. chaffeensis, which causes HME, occurs primarily in the southeastern and south-central United States. The Lone Star tick, *Amblyomma americanum*, serves as the primary vector, while the white-tailed deer is the main reservoir host. As suggested by the disease name, this agent infects human monocytic blood cells; however, despite this intracellular location, *E. chaffeenis* has not been implicated in a transfusion case. Two hundred cases of HME were reported in the United States during the year 2000,[50] but this figure is probably an underestimate of the true number of cases because HME became a notifiable disease only in 1999, with reporting limited to 36 states. *E. chaffeensis* infection also has been reported from patients in Asia, Europe, and Africa, but these reports remain largely unconfirmed.[51-54]

A. phagocytophilum (formerly called *Ehrlichia* sp. or *E. phagocytophila*) is the etiologic agent of HGE and was first described in 1994. The known geographic distribution of this agent is limited to the United States, parts of Europe, and apparently Korea.[52,55] In the United States, the distribution of *A. phagocytophilum* is similar to that of *B. microti*: the Northeast, Upper Midwest, and Pacific Northwest. The similarities in geographic distribution for these two agents are likely attributable to their shared tick vectors: *I. scapularis* in the Northeast and Upper Midwest and apparently *I. pacificus* in the Pacific Northwest. During 2000, 351 cases of HGE were reported in the United States, but as indicated for cases of HME, HGE has only recently become a notifiable disease that is reportable in only a limited number of states.[50] As for *B. divergens*, the European vector for *A. phagocytophilum* is thought to be *I. ricinus*, while a Korean vector has not been identified.

Clinical Symptoms

Similar to other tick-borne diseases (eg, Lyme disease, babesiosis), ehrlichiosis symptoms are generally subclinical or mild, characterized by fever, headache, and general malaise that begins 1 to 3 weeks after infection. About one-third of infections with *E. chaffeensis* also demonstrate a rash, but among cases of HGE, a rash is rare and may not be diagnostic.[55,56] Symptoms associated with more severe cases of ehrlichiosis may include acute renal failure, gastrointestinal bleeding, acute respiratory distress syndrome, and secondary opportunistic infections, with reported fatality rates of up to 5% for HGE and 10% for HME.[51]

Diagnosis and Treatment

During the first week of infection, initial diagnosis of HME and HGE can be accomplished by examining stained peripheral blood smears for the characteristic intracytoplasmic inclusions called morulae.[55] The phenotype of the infected cell (ie, monocyte or neutrophil) is also diagnostic, allowing one to differentiate between infections with *E. chaffeensis* and *A. phagocytophilum*. After the first week, serologic detection by IFA is the most frequently used assay for clinical diagnosis.[57] Sensitive PCR assays for the detection of amplified rickettsial DNA have been developed that are useful for identifying early acute infections.[58,59] Once diagnosed, ehrlichial infections are generally treated with either doxycycline or tetracycline hydrochloride.[51,55]

Seroprevalence

There are few published seroprevalence studies of these ehrlichial agents, probably due to their relatively recent emergence as agents of concern and the limited number of testing options available. In the general population, three studies have reported rates for *A. phagocytophilum*; 0.4% (n = 219) of Northern California residents, 3.4% (n = 671) of New York residents, and 14.9% (n = 475) of Northwestern Wisconsin residents had antibodies to *A. phagocytophilum*.[29,60,61] Two studies have also investigated the seroprevalence rate of *A. phagocytophilum* in blood donors. In the first study, 11.3% (n = 159) of Westchester County (NY) donors had *A. phagocytophilum* antibodies,[62] whereas a second study observed that 0.5% (n = 992) of Wisconsin donors and 3.5% (n = 992) of Connecticut donors had antibodies to *A. phagocytophilum*.[28]

Transfusion Transmission

The only ehrlichial agent thus far implicated in a transfusion-transmitted case is *A. phagocytophilum*. This case involved a patient with rheumatoid arthritis who received two, non-leukocyte-reduced RBC units.[63] Less than 2 weeks after the transfusion, *A. phagocytophilum* was confirmed in the recipient by blood smear, serology (1:512), and PCR. The recipient was subsequently treated with doxycycline and the infection rapidly resolved. The implicated donor was tested by IFA and found to be seropositive for *A. phagocytophilum* at 1:2048. This donor reported a history of Lyme disease and had experienced extensive deer tick bites 2 months before the implicated donation.

Despite the paucity of ehrlichial transfusion cases, the agents of HGE and HME are well suited for transmission by transfusion, given their intracellular location and ability to survive under blood bank conditions. Indeed, *A. phagocytophilum* has been shown to survive in refrigerated blood for up to 18 days.[64] Moreover, in the *A. phagocytophilum* transmission case described above, the implicated RBC unit was 30 days old, suggesting that the agent may survive and remain viable over a longer period.[63] While no transfusion cases have been reported for *E. chaffeensis*, the agent has been shown to remain viable in ADSOL-treated RBC units stored at 4 to 6 C for at least 11 days.[65]

Control Strategies

Given that *E. chaffeensis* and *A. phagocytophilum* pose a minimal transfusion threat at this time, it may seem premature to consider strategies to prevent their transmission. However, as the endemic range of these agents expands and clinical cases become more widely recognized, the number of transfusion cases is likely to increase. Much of the discussion concerning control of *Babesia* spp. transmission is applicable to *E. chaffeensis* and *A. phagocytophilum*. Deferral strategies based on donor-reported tick bites are counterproductive. Similarly, donors reporting tick bites do not appear to be at a greater risk for infection with *A. phagocytophilum* than control donors.[28] This observation is interesting because, unlike *Babesia* spp., *A.*

phagocytophilum can be transmitted by ticks that have fed for only 24 hours.[66]

Testing strategies for *E. chaffeensis* and *A. phagocytophilum* are limited by a general lack of suitable tests. For both agents, the primary serologic test is the IFA, which is generally assembled in-house or purchased through commercial manufacturers. Research-based PCR assays have also been developed,[58,59] and as already discussed, these may be useful for defining window period infections.

In addition to testing, leukocyte reduction may also offer some level of enhanced blood safety. Studies conducted using another rickettsial agent, *O. tsutsugamuchi*, demonstrated a 10^5 reduction in the number of infectious rickettsia in a mouse model.[67] In contrast, *E. chaffeensis* has been reisolated from the supernatant fraction of leukocyte-reduced RBCs.[65] Taken together, leukocyte reduction may filter out cells that contain intracellular riskettsia but fail to remove those that are extracellular.

Preliminary studies with pathogen inactivation agents suggest that rickettsial agents may be susceptible to psoralen compounds. Again, these studies used mononuclear cells infected with the scrub typhus agent *O. tsutsugamuchi* that were inoculated into platelet concentrates.[68] Subsequently, psoralen-treated platelets were injected into mice, which demonstrated no signs of infection with *O. tsutsugamuchi*, whereas control mice rapidly became ill and/or died.

Other Agents

Several other parasitic agents are either potentially transmissible by blood transfusion or have been implicated in a transfusion case. For the most part, transfusion cases involving these agents are extremely rare despite long-term surveillance of them. This chapter has primarily focused on tick-borne agents, especially those transmitted by *Ixodes* ticks. It is perhaps surprising that a transfusion case involving *Borrelia burgdorferi*, the agent of Lyme disease, has never been reported, despite being found in the same ticks as *B. microti* and *A. phagocytophilum*. Moreover, because innumerable cases of Lyme disease have been reported in the United States, Europe, and other parts of the world, one would have anticipated that a transfusion case would have been identified if the agent was readily transmitted. Occasionally, blood donors are diagnosed with Lyme disease a few days after donating blood, but attempts to identify the agent in recipients receiving their blood have been unsuccessful.[69] One could infer that *B. burgdorferi* does not survive under blood storage conditions. However, laboratory studies indicate that *B. burgdorferi* survives under frozen, refrigerated, or 20 to 24 C storage conditions for the duration of the storage period of Fresh Frozen Plasma, RBCs, and Platelets, respectively.[70]

Several explanations have been offered for the lack of *B. burgdorferi* transfusion cases. First, it is unlikely that most cases of transfusion-transmitted *B. burgdorferi* would be recognized by physicians due to the nonspecific nature of Lyme disease symptoms. Second, the characteristic lesion or erythema migrans, which often appears in association with the tick bite, is unlikely to be present following the intravenous injection of spirochetes during blood transfusion.[71] Last, because it has been difficult to demonstrate spirochetes in patients with active Lyme disease,[72] the spirochetemic phase may be very short, thus diminishing the likelihood of successful transmission by transfusion. Despite the lack of observed transfusion cases, continued surveillance of this agent is warranted.

In contrast, another tick-borne agent, *Rickettsia rickettsia*, has been implicated in a transfusion transmission case. *R. rickettsia* is a rickettsial agent that causes Rocky Mountain Spotted Fever (RMSF), the most common fatal tick-borne disease in the United States. This agent is limited to the Western Hemisphere, causing RMSF in North America and a similar disease, Brazilian Spotted Fever, in South America. The transfusion case involved a donor who developed symptomatic RMSF 3 days after donation and died several days later.[73] *R. rickettsia* infection of the recipient was confirmed by serology, cell culture, and animal inoculation. The recipient was treated for RMSF and had an uneventful recovery.

Two protozoan parasites, *Toxoplasma gondii* and *Leishmania* spp., have been transmitted by blood transfusion on several occasions, although few contemporary cases have been reported.[74] The lack of more frequent transfusion cases involving these agents is somewhat surprising, considering the incidence rates for these agents in human populations. A recent US study reported that 22.5% of people tested in a large survey (n = 17,658) demonstrated antibodies to *T. gondii*,[75] whereas the seroprevalence rates for *T. gondii* in other parts of the world are reportedly much higher. As for *Leishmania* infection, approximately 350 million people worldwide are at risk for infection and 2 million new cases of leishmaniasis are estimated to occur each year.[76] Further, tachyzoites of *T. gondii* have been reported to remain viable in blood components stored at 4 C for up to 50 days after collection.[77] Likewise, studies with *L. tropica* and *L. donovani* indicate that *Leishmania* parasites contained within infected mononuclear cells remain viable for 25 days in RBC units and for at least 5 days in platelets maintained under blood bank conditions.[78] The limited number of transfusion cases attributable to these agents may be the result of the short parasitemic phase exhibited by *T. gondii* and the intermittent and low density with which *Leishmania* parasites circulate in an infected host.[79]

The last group of parasitic agents that may be transmitted by blood transfusion are those that cause filariasis. Unlike most helminth infections in humans, filarial infections have a distinct and ongoing phase of their life cycle during which sufficient numbers of larval stages (ie, microfilariae) are present in peripheral blood to pose a threat to blood safety. Those filariae of primary concern to blood safety are *Wuchereria bancrofti* and *Brugia malayi,* which cause elephantiasis in the lower extremities, and *Loa loa*, which migrates through subcutaneous tissue causing localized inflammation. Studies have shown that microfilariae are capable of surviving in refrigerated blood for up to 21 days.[80,81] Taken together, one would expect transmission of these agents by blood transfusion to occur with some regularity. However, before microfilariae can progress to the infective filariform stage, they must pass through several molts within a vector. Thus, microfilariae introduced from a donor to a recipient are incapable of maturing to adulthood. For this reason, transmission of filariae by transfusion should be relatively benign and likely go undetected, with the exception of an immunologic reaction to dying microfilariae.

Summary

Parasitic agents, along with viruses and bacteria, pose significant risks to blood safety. Among parasitic agents, *Plasmodium* spp. and *T. cruzi* have historically garnered most of the attention whether through surveillance, epidemiologic studies, or, in the case of *Plasmodium* spp., implementation of control measures. The relatively recent emergence of other parasitic agents, particularly those transmitted by ticks, indicates that blood safety issues posed by these agents need to be addressed as well. Foremost among these agents is *B. microti,* which has been implicated in an ever-increasing number of transfusion cases while its known endemic range continues to expand. Other more recently emerged agents such as *A. phagocytophilum* require continued surveillance and implementation of epidemiologic studies designed to determine the likelihood of their transmission by blood transfusion. One can be assured that these will not be the last parasitic agents to pose a threat to blood safety, as other agents will continue to emerge in the near future.

References

1. Kjemtrup AM, Conrad PA. Human babesiosis: An emerging tick-borne disease. Int J Parasitol 2000;30:1323-37.
2. Scholtens RG, Braff EH, Healy GR, Gleason N. A case of babesiosis in man in the United States. Am J Trop Med Hyg 1968;17:810-13.

3. McQuiston JH, Childs JE, Chamberland ME, et al. Transmission of tick-borne agents by blood transfusion: A review of known and potential risks in the United States. Transfusion 2000;40:274-84.
4. White DJ, Talarico J, Chang H-G, et al. Human babesiosis in New York State. Review of 139 hospitalized cases and analysis of prognostic factors. Arch Intern Med 1998;158:2149-54.
5. Herwaldt BL, McGovern PC, Gerwel MP, et al. Endemic babesiosis in another eastern state: New Jersey. Emerg Infect Dis 2003;9:184-8.
6. Quick RE, Herwaldt BL, Thromford JW, et al. Babesiosis in Washington State: A new species of *Babesia*? Ann Intern Med 1993;119:284-90.
7. Persing DH, Herwaldt BL, Glaser C, et al. Infection with a *Babesia*-like organism in northern California. N Engl J Med 1995;332:298-303.
8. Herwaldt BL, Persing DH, Précigout EA, et al. A fatal case of babesiosis in Missouri: Identification of another piroplasm that infects humans. Ann Intern Med 1996;124:643-50.
9. Beattie JF, Michelson ML, Holman PJ. Acute babesiosis caused by *Babesia divergens* in a resident of Kentucky. N Engl J Med 2002;347: 697-8.
10. Homer MJ, Aguilar-Delfin I, Telfored SR, et al. Babesiosis. Clin Microbiol Rev 2000;13:451-69.
11. Gorenflot A, Moubri K, Précigout E, et al. Human babesiosis. Ann Trop Med Parasitol 1998;92:489-501.
12. Saito-Ito A, Tsuji M, Wei Q, et al. Transfusion-acquired, autochthonous human babesiosis in Japan: Isolation of *Babesia microti*-like parasites with hu-RBC-SCID mice. J Clin Microbiol 2000;38:4511-6.
13. Piesman J, Spielman A. *Babesia microti*: Infectivity of parasites from ticks for hamsters and white-footed mice. Exp Parasitol 1982;53:242-8.
14. Meldrum SC, Birkhead GS, White DJ, et al. Human babesiosis in New York State: An epidemiologic description of 136 cases. Clin Infect Dis 1992;15:1019-23.
15. Sun T, Tenenbaum MJ, Greenspan J, et al. Morphologic and clinical observations in human infection with *Babesia microti*. J Infect Dis 1983; 148:239-48.
16. Chisholm ES, Ruebush TK, Sulzer AJ, Healy GR. *Babesia microti* infection in man: Evaluation of an indirect immunofluorescent antibody test. Am J Trop Med Hyg 1978;27:14-9.
17. Houghton RL, Homer MJ, Reynolds LD, et al. Identification of *Babesia microti*-specific immunodominant epitopes and development of a peptide EIA for detection of antibodies in serum. Transfusion 2002;42: 1488-96.
18. Persing DH, Mathiesen D, Marshall WF, et al. Detection of *Babesia microti* by polymerase chain reaction. J Clin Microbiol 1992;30:2097-103.
19. Olmeda AS, Armstrong PM, Rosenthal BM, et al. A subtropical case of human babesiosis. Acta Trop 1997;67:229-34.
20. Herwaldt BL, Kjemtrup AM, Conrad PA, et al. Transfusion-transmitted babesiosis in Washington state: First reported case caused by a WA1-type parasite. J Infect Dis 1997;175:1259-62.

21. Krause PJ, Spielman A, Telford SR, et al. Persistent parasitemia after acute babesiosis. N Engl J Med 1998;339:160-4.
22. Krause PJ, Lepore T, Sikand VK, et al. Atovaquone and azithromycin for the treatment of babesiosis. N Engl J Med 2000;343:1454-8.
23. Machtinger L, Telford SR, Inducil C, et al. Treatment of babesiosis by red blood cell exchange in an HIV-positive, splenectomized patient. J Clin Apheresis 1993;8:78-81.
24. Dorman SE, Cannon ME, Telford SR, et al. Fulminant babesiosis treated with clindamycin, quinine, and whole-blood exchange transfusion. Transfusion 2000;40:375-80.
25. Pantanowitz L, Telford SR, Cannon ME. The impact of babesiosis on transfusion medicine. Transfus Med Rev 2002;16:131-43.
26. Popovsky MA, Lindberg LE, Syrek AL, Page PL. Prevalence of *Babesia* antibody in a selected blood donor population. Transfusion 1988;28: 59-61.
27. Linden JV, Wong SJ, Chu FK, et al. Transfusion-associated transmission of babesiosis in New York State. Transfusion 2000;40:285-9.
28. Leiby DA, Chung APS, Cable RG, et al. Relationship between tick bites and the seroprevalence of *Babesia microti* and *Anaplasma phagocytophila* (previously *Ehrlichia* sp.) in blood donors. Transfusion 2002;42:1585-91.
29. Fritz CL, Kjemtrup AM, Conrad PA, et al. Seroepidemiology of emerging tickborne infectious diseases in a Northern California community. J Infect Dis 1997;175:1432-9.
30. Lux JZ, Weiss D, Linden JV, et al. Transfusion-associated babesiosis after heart transplant. Emerg Infect Dis 2003;9:116-9.
31. Matsui T, Inoue R, Kajimoto K, et al. First documentation of transfusion-associated babesiosis in Japan [article in Japanese with English summary]. Rinsho Ketsueki 2000;41:628-34.
32. Jassoum BS, Fong IW, Hannach B, et al. Transfusion-transmitted babesiosis in Ontario: First reported case in Canada. Can Commun Dis Rep 2000;26:9-13.
33. Kjemtrup AM, Lee B, Fritz CL, et al. Investigation of transfusion transmission of a WA1-type babesial parasite to a premature infant in California. Transfusion 2002;42:1482-7.
34. Gerber MA, Shapiro ED, Krause PJ, et al. The risk of acquiring Lyme disease or babesiosis from a blood transfusion. J Infect Dis 1994;170; 231-4.
35. Cable RG, Badon S, Trouern-Trend J, et al. Evidence for transmission of *Babesia microti* from Connecticut blood donors to recipients (abstract). Transfusion 2001;41(Suppl):12S-13S.
36. Mintz ED, Anderson JF, Cable RG, Hadler JL. Transfusion-transmitted babesiosis: A case report from a new endemic area. Transfusion 1991; 31:365-8.
37. Eberhard ML, Walker EM, Steurer FJ. Survival and infectivity of *Babesia* in blood maintained at 25 C and 2-4 C. J Parasitol 1995;81:790-2.

38. Strle F, Nadelman RB, Cimperman J, et al. Comparison of culture-confirmed erythema migrans caused by *Borrelia burgdorferi* sensu stricto in New York State and by *Borrelia afzellii* in Slovenia. Ann Intern Med 1999;130:32-6.
39. White DJ, Talarico J, Chang H, et al. Human babesiosis in New York State. Review of 139 hospitalized cases and analysis of prognostic factors. Arch Intern Med 1998;158:2149-54.
40. Fishbein DB, Dawson JE, Robinson LA. Human ehrlichiosis in the United States, 1985 to 1990. Ann Intern Med 1994;120:736-43.
41. Grellier P, Santus R, Louray E, et al. Photosensitized inactivation of *Plasmodium falciparum*- and *Babesia divergens*-infected erythrocytes in whole blood by lipophilic pheophorbide derivatives. Vox Sang 1997; 72:211-20.
42. Misao T, Koboyashi Y. Studies on infectious mononucleosis: Isolation of etiologic agent from blood, bone marrow, and lymph node of a patient with infectious mononucleosis by using mice. Tokyo Iji Shinshi 1954;71:683-6.
43. Perez M, Rikihisa Y, Wen B. *Ehrlichia canis*-like agent isolated from a man in Venezuela: Antigenic and genetic characterization. J Clin Microbiol 1996;34:2133-9.
44. Buller RS, Arens M, Hmiel SP, et al. *Ehrlichia ewingii*, a newly recognized agent of human ehrlichiosis. N Engl J Med 1999;341:148-55.
45. Maeda K, Markowitz N, Hawley RC, et al. Human infection with *Ehrlichia canis*, a leukocytic rickettsia. N Engl J Med 1987;316:853-6.
46. Anderson BE, Dawson JE, Jones DC, Wilson KH. *Ehrlichia chaffeensis*, a new species associated with human ehrlichiosis. J Clin Microbiol 1991; 29:2838-42.
47. Bakken JS, Dumler JS, Chen S-M, et al. Human granulocytic erhlichiosis in the Upper Midwest United States. A new species emerging? JAMA 1994;272:212-8.
48. Chen S-M, Dumler SJ, Bakken JS, Walker DH. Identification of a granulocytic *Ehrlichia* species as the etiologic agent of human disease. J Clin Microbiol 1994;32:589-95.
49. Dumler JS, Barbet AF, Bekker CPJ, et al. Reorganization of genera in the families *Rickettsiaceae* and *Anaplasmataceae* in the order *Rickettsiales*: Unification of some species of *Ehrlichia* with *Anaplasma*, *Cowdria* with *Ehrlichia* and *Ehrlichia* with *Neorickettsia*, descriptions of six new species combinations and designation of *Ehrlichia equi* and "HGE agent" as subjective synonyms of *Ehrlichia phagocytophila*. Int J Syst Evol Microbiol 2001;51:2145-65.
50. Centers for Disease Control and Prevention. Summary of notifiable diseases—United States, 2000. MMWR Morb Mortal Wkly Rep 2002; 49:x-xi.
51. Dumler JS, Bakken JS. Ehrlichial diseases of humans: Emerging tick-borne infections. Clin Infect Dis 1995;20:1102-10.
52. Heo E-J, Park J-H, Koo J-R, et al. Serologic and molecular detection of *Ehrlichia chaffeensis* and *Anaplasma phagocytophila* (human

granulocytic ehrlichiosis agent) in Korean patients. J Clin Microbiol 2002;40:3082-5.
53. Keysary A, Amram L, Keren G, et al. Serologic evidence of human monocytic and granulocytic ehrlichiosis in Israel. Emerg Infect Dis 1999;5:775-8.
54. Brouqui P, Dumler JS. Serologic evidence of human monocytic and granulocytic ehrlichiosis in Israel (letter). Emerg Infect Dis 2000;6:314.
55. Bakken JS, Dumler JS. Human granulocytic ehrlichiosis. Clin Infect Dis 2000;31:554-60.
56. Fritz CL, Glaser CA. Ehrlichiosis. Infect Dis Clin North Am 1998; 341:148-55.
57. Walls JJ, Aguero-Rosenfeld M, Bakken JS, et al. Inter- and intralaboratory comparison of *Ehrlichia equi* and human granulocytic ehrlichiosis (HGE) agent strains for serodiagnosis of HGE by immunofluorescent-antibody test. J Clin Microbiol 1999;37:2968-73.
58. Everett ED, Evans KA, Henry RB, McDonald G. Human ehrlichiosis in adults after tick exposure. Diagnosis using polymerase chain reaction. Ann Intern Med 1994;120:730-5.
59. Massung RF, Slater K, Owens JH, et al. Nested PCR assay for detection of granulocytic ehrlichiae. J Clin Microbiol 1998;36:1090-5.
60. Hilton E, DeVoti J, Benach JL, et al. Seroprevalence and seroconversion for tick-borne diseases in a high-risk population in the northeast United States. Am J Med 1999;106:404-9.
61. Bakken JS, Goellner P, Van Etten M, et al. Seroprevalence of human granulocytic ehrlichiosis among permanent residents of northwestern Wisconsin. Clin Infect Dis 1998;27:1491-6.
62. Aguero-Rosenfeld ME, Donnarumma L, Zentmaier L, et al. Seroprevalence of antibodies that react with *Anaplasma phagocytophila*, the agent of human granulocytic ehrlichiosis, in different populations in Westchester County, New York. J Clin Microbiol 2002;40:2612-5.
63. Eastlund T, Persing D, Mathiesen D, et al. Human granulocytic ehrlichiosis after red cell transfusion (abstract). Transfusion 1999;39 (Suppl):117S.
64. Kalantarpour F, Chowdhury I, Wormser GP, et al. Survival of the human granulocytic ehrlichiosis agent under refrigeration conditions. J Clin Microbiol 2000;38:2398-9.
65. McKechnie DB, Slater KS, Childs JE, et al. Survival of *Ehrlichia chaffeensis* in refrigerated, ADSOL-treated RBCs. Transfusion 2000;40:1041-7.
66. des Vignes F, Piesman J, Heffernan R, et al. Effect of tick removal on transmission of *Borrelia burgdorferi* and *Anaplasma phagocytophila* by *Ixodes scapularis* nymphs. J Infect Dis 2001;183:773-8.
67. Mettille FC, Salata KF, Belanger KJ, et al. Reducing the risk of transfusion-transmitted rickettsial disease by WBC filtration, using *Orientia tsutsugamushi* in a model system. Transfusion 2000;40:290-6.
68. Belanger KJ, Kelly DJ, Mettille FC, et al. Psoralen photochemical inactivation or *Orientia tsutsugamushi* in platelet concentrates. Transfusion 2000;40:1503-7.

69. Cable R, Krause P, Badon S, et al. Acute blood donor co-infection with *Babesia microti* (Bm) and *Borrelia burgdorferi* (Bb) (abstract). Transfusion 1993;33(Suppl):50S.
70. Badon SJ, Fister RD, Cable RG. Survival of *Borrelia burgdorferi* in blood products. Transfusion 1989;29:581-3.
71. Cable RG, Trouern-Trend J. Tickborne infections. In: Linden JV, Bianco C, eds. Blood safety and surveillance. New York: Marcel Dekker, 2001: 399-422.
72. Shrestha M, Grodzicki RL, Steere AC. Diagnosing early Lyme disease. Am J Med 1985;78:235-40.
73. Randall WH, Simmons J, Casper EA, Philip RN. Transmission of Colorado tick fever virus by blood transfusion—Montana. MMWR Morb Mortal Wkly Rep 1975;24:422-7.
74. Dodd RY. Transmission of parasites by blood transfusion. Vox Sang 1998;74(Suppl 2):161-3.
75. Jones JL, Kruszon-Moran D, Wilson M, et al. *Toxoplasma gondii* infection in the United States: Seroprevalence and risk factors. Am J Epidemiol 2001;154:357-65.
76. Herwaldt BL. Leishmaniasis. Lancet 1999;354:1191-9.
77. Talice RV, Gurri J, Royol J, Prez-Moreira L. Investigaciones sobre la toxoplasmosis en el Uraguay. Sobrevida de *Toxoplasma gondii* en sangre humana "in vitro." Ann Fac Med Montey 1957;42:143-7.
78. Grogl M, Daugirda JL, Hoover DL, et al. Survivability and infectivity of viscerotropic *Leishmania tropica* from Operation Desert Storm participants in human blood products maintained under blood bank conditions. Am J Trop Med Hyg 1993;49:308-15.
79. Le Fichoux Y, Quaranta J-M, Aufeuvre J-P, et al. Occurrence of *Leishmania infantum* parasitemia in asymptomatic blood donors living in an area of endemicity in southern France. J Clin Microbiol 1999;37: 1953-7.
80. AuBuchon JP, Dzik WH. Survival of *Loa loa* in banked blood. Lancet 1983;1:647-8.
81. Bird GWG, Menon KK. Survival of *Microfilaria bancrofti* in stored blood. Lancet 1961;ii:721.

In: Brecher ME, ed.
Bacterial and Parasitic Contamination of Blood Components
Bethesda, MD: AABB Press, 2003

9

Pathogen Inactivation Methods

STEPHEN J. WAGNER, PHD

OVER THE PAST THREE DECADES, NUMEROUS donor screening and infectious disease testing methods have been implemented to reduce the transmission of human immunodeficiency virus (HIV), hepatitis C virus (HCV), hepatitis B virus (HBV), and human T-cell lymphotropic viruses I and II (HTLV-I/II). As a result, the residual risk of virus transmission in blood components has declined to approximately 1 in 2,000,000 for HIV, 1 in 2,000,000 for HCV, 1 in 250,000 for HBV, and 1 in 250,000 to 2,000,000 for HTLV-I/ II.[1-3] Although the viral safety of the blood supply has

---

Stephen J. Wagner, PhD, Director, Cell Therapy Development, Blood and Cell Therapy Development, American Red Cross Biomedical Research and Development, Rockville, Maryland

increased dramatically with the adoption of donor screening and testing measures, the risks of bacterial sepsis and parasite infection have remained unchanged. On the basis of the available evidence, roughly 17% of transfusion-related fatalities reported to the Food and Drug Administration (FDA) between 1978 to 1998 have been caused by bacterial contamination; these septic fatalities represent the greatest infectious disease risk among transfusion fatalities.[4] The risk is greatest from platelet transfusions, with 1 in 60,000 units[5] to 1 in 450,000 units[6] transfused resulting in fatalities. In addition, there is increasing recognition that parasites other than malaria, such as *Babesia microti* and *Trypanosoma cruzi*, can be transmitted by blood in the United States.[7-11] Although fewer data are available, the risk of transmission of these agents may be as great as or greater than those associated with the current viral risks for tested agents.

With the reduction of viral risk, the risks of sepsis and parasite infection have taken on increased relative importance. Development of new infectious disease tests and pathogen reduction methods represent two alternative approaches to reduce transfusion-transmitted bacteria and parasite infections. In addition, pathogen inactivation may provide an additional layer of safety to reduce the residual risk from tested viruses and may potentially reduce the transmission of unrecognized or uncharacterized blood-borne agents. This chapter reviews the recent progress in developing methods for bacterial and parasite reduction of cellular blood components.

Bacteria and Parasite Reduction Methods in Red Cells

Frangible Anchor Linker Effector (FRALE) Alkylating Agents

FRALE compounds are patterned after the alkylating agent, quinacrine mustard (Fig 9-1).[12,13] Quinacrine mustard consists of a planar acridine ring (which serves as an anchor and intercalates between nucleic acid bases), a nitrogen mustard

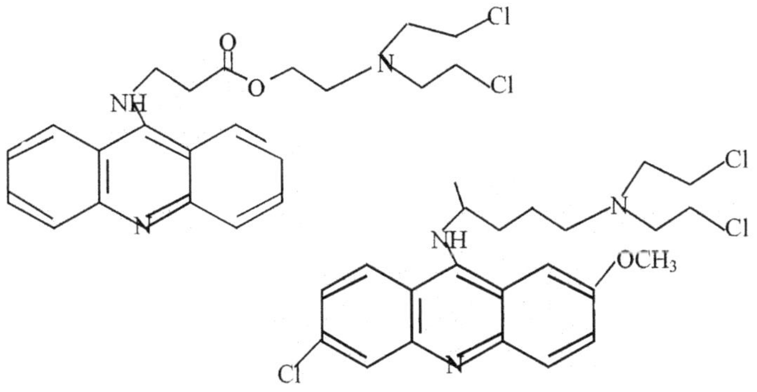

Figure 9-1. Structure of S-303 (left) and quinacrine mustard (right).

effector (which forms covalent adducts and crosslinks with nucleic acid bases), and an alkyl linker (which joins the anchor and effector portions of the molecule). Nucleic acid adducts and crosslinks prevent polymerase passage across the lesions and thus prevent pathogen replication. Red cells, which do not contain nucleic acid, are relatively unaffected by FRALE treatment (see below). The linker region in FRALE compounds contains a frangible ester bond that is cleaved at a rate slower than adduct formation in blood components. The cleavage of the linker group does not interfere with pathogen inactivation but provides a means to break down unreacted FRALE compound into a negatively charged product that is not expected to further interact with nucleic acids. An example of the FRALE compound, S-303, is given in Fig 9-1.

Investigators have used 150 μM S-303 to inactivate a number of viruses during 2-hour room temperature incubation.[14] Under virucidal conditions, high levels of bacteria inactivation were demonstrated: >7 log *Yersinia enterocolitica;* 4.8 log *Salmonella typhimurium;* >7.4 log *Escherichia coli;* >7 log *Listeria monocytogenes;* 5.2 log *Staphylococcus epidermidis;* >6 log *Deinococcus radiodurans.* No published studies on parasite inactivation with S-303 are available.

Red cell in-vitro properties and function are well preserved after S-303 treatment. Adenosine triphosphate, 2,3-diphosphoglycerate, glucose, and lactose levels are comparable after treated and control units are stored at 1 to 6 C for up to 42 days.[15] The rate of potassium leakage from S-303-treated red cells stored at 1 to 6 C is very similar to control red cells. There is, however, some evidence that FRALE treatment has the potential to alter the red cell surface. Flow cytometry studies using a fluorescently labeled antibody directed against the acridine moiety of another FRALE compound, PIC-1, suggest that FRALE compounds react with the red cell surface.[16] These red cell surface reactions can be greatly reduced by the addition of millimolar levels of glutathione to the treatment procedure. Presumably, glutathione acts as an extracellular quencher of FRALE to prevent reactions to red cell surface proteins. The addition of glutathione does not change appreciably the antiviral activity of FRALE compounds. However, no published data are available to ascertain whether S-303 treatment causes a reduction of intracellular glutathione levels in red cells. Red cell experiments with S-303-treated and control cells stored for 35 days at 1 to 6 C before autologous infusion indicate good 24-hour recovery, with values of 83.9 ± 6.05% for the control group and 78.7 ± 5.69% for the treated group.[17] In a second clinical trial, the subjects who received S-303-treated and control red cells in the first trial received five additional infusions of S-303-treated red cells over a 35-day period, with administration of radiolabeled S-303 red cells at day 35.[18] For the control group, which subsequently received S-303 red cells, the 24-hour recovery was 84.2 ± 6.4%, and the 24-hour recovery of the S-303 group, which subsequently received S-303 red cells, was 78.1 ± 6.1%.

Quinacrine mustard, which has structural similarities to S-303 (Fig 9-1), is highly mutagenic in the Ames test using nanomolar concentrations of the compound (TA1537 tester strain).[12] Similar findings of genotoxicity with quinacrine mustard have been demonstrated in the mouse lymphoma-forward mutation assay and in the sister chromatid exchange assay using human cells.[19,20] However, quinacrine mustard breaks down in red cell suspensions with prolonged incubation; red cells incubated overnight with quinacrine mustard concentrations from 0.3 to 3 μM displayed no mutagenic activity in the Ames test. Removal of residual quinacrine mustard or its breakdown products with an Amberlite XAD-16 resin from red cell samples incubated overnight with 0.3 to 10 μM compound also demonstrated no discernible mutagenic activity.

Additional studies have focused on genotoxicity studies of S-303 following treatment of red cells.[21]. Treatment conditions were defined as 0.2 mM S-303 in red cells, followed by 24-hour room temperature incubation. Red cell samples treated in this manner were negative in the Ames test, the chromosome aberration assay, and the micronucleus test. Further studies using transgenic p53 mice infused thrice weekly for 26 weeks with incubated red cells that were previously treated with 1 mM S-303 indicated that there were no test-article-induced toxicities or carcinogenicities observed. No studies have been published on the genotoxicity or carcinogenicity of S-303 before its addition to red cells.

INACTINE Compounds

INACTINE compounds are patterned after the nucleic acid alkylating agent, ethylenimine (Fig 9-2). INACTINES consist of a planar, three-member aziridine ring joined to an alkyl chain containing a repeating, positively charged amine.[22] INACTINE forms nucleic acid adducts that prevent polymerase from traversing the lesion and therefore inhibit pathogen nucleic acid replication. The aziridine group is responsible for the alkylating activity; the repeating positive charges on the alkyl chain presumably promote interaction with the negatively charged phosphate backbone on nucleic acids. Specific-

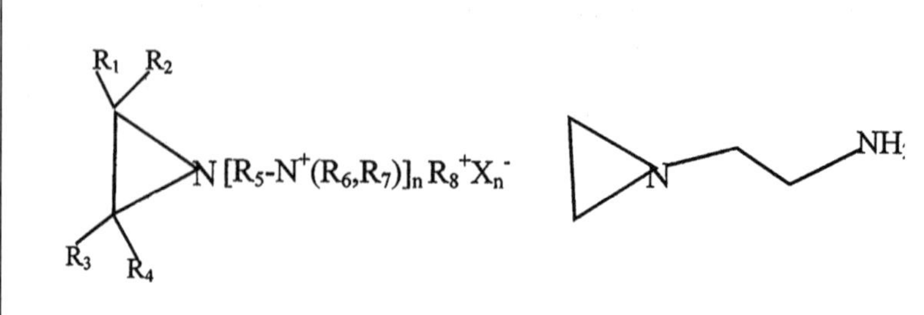

Figure 9-2. Generic structure of INACTINES (left) and structure of ethylenimine (right).

ity for nucleic acid has been demonstrated by a lack of reactivity to viral proteins.[23,24] Despite the specificity to nucleic acids, some amino acids such as cysteine and some proteins such as lysozyme react with ethylenimine.[25,26]

Investigators have used room temperature incubation of 0.1% (v/v) of the INACTINE, PEN110, with red cell suspensions for pathogen reduction. Using deliberately inoculated units of red cells containing 10 to 100 CFU/mL of *Y. enterocolitica, Pseudomonas fluorescens,* or *Pseudomonas putida,* treatment of PEN110 for 24 hours resulted in no subsequent bacterial growth during 42-day 1 to 6 C storage, with all samples containing no detectable bacteria.[27] Heavy bacterial outgrowth was evident in all control units, which were immediately stored at 1 to 6 C after inoculation. However, four of 15 experiments that involved sham addition of PEN110 with 24-hour room temperature storage before refrigerated storage resulted in no bacterial growth, suggesting the presence of temperature-dependent antibacterial factors in red cell suspensions. Given the contribution of blood elements as well as PEN110 to antibacterial activity, it is difficult to predict the actual level of pathogen reduction in these experiments. Nevertheless, assuming that *no* blood-derived antibacterial factors were present in 300 mL units, the upper limit of bacterial inactivation in this system is calculated to be between 3.5 to 4.5 log. In another series of experiments using greater inoculum levels of 10^4 CFU/mL, *Y. enterocolitica* or *P. fluorescens* outgrowth was evident in two of three units within 2 weeks after PEN110 treatment.[28] These results suggest that the PEN110 treatment was not able to completely inactivate high levels (>10^4 CFU/mL) of these organisms.

Experiments have been described demonstrating the inactivation of *T. cruzi* trypomastigotes by PEN110 in heat-inactivated supernatant derived from red cells containing additive solution.[29] *T. cruzi* trypomastigotes were deliberately contaminated in the diluted plasma and incubated with 0.001, 0.005, 0.01, 0.05, and 0.1% PEN110 for 1 or 3 hours at room temperature and subsequently washed to remove the residual drug. Washed treated and control samples were used to infect Vero cell monolayers and subsequently analyzed by microscopic evaluation. For each concentration, >1500 Vero cells were observed for signs of infection. The number of infected cells and swimming parasites were decreased greater than 10-fold in samples containing 0.001% PEN110. No infected cells were observed with PEN110 concentrations ≥0.005%. It is unknown whether these results in diluted plasma could be extended to red cell suspensions.

Investigators have explored whether PEN110 treatment inactivates *B. microti* in red cells.[30] Parasite-infected human and hamster red cells (inoculum titer was not stated) were either used as controls or treated with 0.01 to 0.1% PEN110 for 24 hours at room temperature. Samples were subsequently assayed for evidence of infection by intraperitoneal inoculation into hamsters. Infection was monitored by blood smear microscopy and by the ability of polymerase chain reaction (PCR) to amplify the *B. microti* template. All concentrations of PEN110 tested inactivated the challenge inoculum of blood infected with *B. microti* to the limit of detection.

Red cell in-vitro properties were affected by 0.1% PEN110 treatment for 4 hours at room temperature, followed by washing in 0.9% saline and resuspension in AS-3 containing 0.2 mM sodium thiosulfate.[31] Hemolysis was elevated in treated samples compared with controls after 42 days of 1 to 6 C storage ($0.7 \pm 0.24\%$ vs $0.23 \pm 0.11\%$, $p<0.05$). The rate of glucose consumption of treated samples was greater than controls over the 42-day storage period [0.37 ± 0.09 vs 0.26 ± 0.09 mmol/10^6 red cells, $p<0.05$ (unpaired t test)]. Similarly, the rate of lactose production of treated samples was greater than controls (0.91 ± 0.012 vs 0.42 ± 0.09 mmole/10^6 red cells, $p<0.05$). A 0.5% decrease of pH was noted in treated samples that was evident after the washing procedure and persisted throughout 42 days of storage. Immediately after PEN110 treatment and washing, concentrations of 2,3-DPG in treated units were reduced by 45% compared to controls ($p<0.05$). Red cell typing remained unchanged in treated units, and direct antiglobulin test results were negative throughout storage.

Two clinical studies have been performed investigating in-vivo red cell 24-hour recovery and survival following PEN110 treatment. In the first study, red cells from 12 normal subjects were exposed to 0.1% PEN110 for 6 hours at room temperature before extensive washing and subsequent quenching of PEN110 with thiosulfate.[31] The residual level of PEN110 was <50 ng/mL. Blood was stored for 28 days, radiolabeled, and 10 mL of either PEN110-treated or control blood was infused autologously in a crossover design. The 24-hour recovery of treated blood was similar to untreated controls ($85.4 \pm 3.5\%$ vs $85.8 \pm 4.2\%$; $p>0.05$). In contrast, the half-life of treated red cells was significantly less than controls [28.5 ± 4.3 days vs 33.5 ± 4.2 days, $p = 0.0089$ (unpaired t test)]. In a second clinical trial, red cells from 24 normal subjects were treated with 0.1% PEN110 for longer room temperature incubation and, thus, more stringent conditions than the first study (24 hours rather than 6 hours).[32] Treated units were extensively washed with an automated cell washer and stored for 35 or 42 days at 1 to 6 C. Aliquots of treated or control samples were radiolabeled, and 10 mL volumes were autologously infused using a crossover design. Results indicated that the 24-hour recovery of PEN110 cells stored up to 42 days was comparable to controls (82.9 ± 5.7 vs 86.3 ± 8.7, p>0.05). No red cell half-life data from this clinical trial have been published to date.

Genotoxicity testing of other aziridines has revealed the potential for mutagenesis, sister chromatid exchanges, and the induction of micronuclei.[33-35] For the aziridine PEN110, acute toxicity testing in New Zealand white rabbits has been reported.[36] Rabbit red cells were treated with 0.1% PEN110 for 24 hours and infused, without washing, into male and female animals to achieve a target PEN110 dose of 3 mg/kg. No evidence of acute toxicity was noted. In a reproductive toxicity investigation, PEN110 was administered intravenously to male and female rats at doses up to 0.5 mg/kg every other day for 2 weeks, subsequently mated, and female rats were similar dosed with PEN110 for the first 16 days of gestation.[37] There was no evidence that PEN110 caused any effects on male or female reproductive function, nor was there any evidence of embryonic toxicity.

Bacteria and Pathogen Reduction Methods in Platelets

Riboflavin and Light

Investigators have taken advantage of the photodynamic properties of vitamin B12, or riboflavin (Fig 9-3), for pathogen reduction in platelet components. Riboflavin can intercalate between nucleic acid bases and, in the presence of either ultraviolet A (UVA) light or blue light, can act as a photosensitizer, producing oxygen-mediated nucleic acid damage.[38,39] Alternatively, illuminated riboflavin can form adducts to DNA by directly reacting with thymine or adenine.[40] Although riboflavin and light treatment can produce nucleic-acid-specific damage, proteins and membranes can be affected as well. Several investigators have reported that riboflavin and light caused enhanced hemolysis in red cells[41,42]; other studies demonstrated riboflavin adducts to serum albumin and eye lens proteins following phototreatment.[43,44]

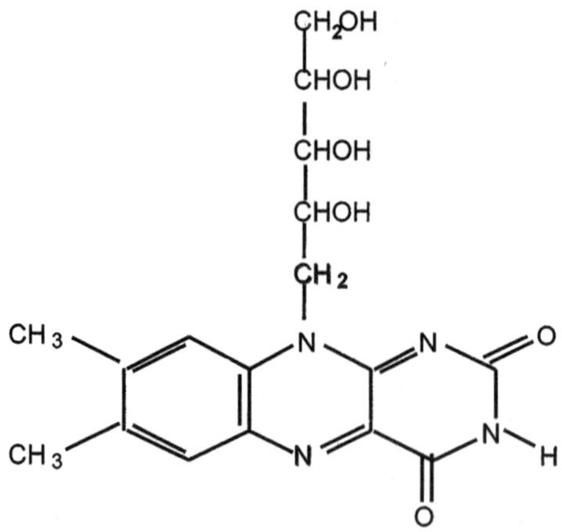

Figure 9-3. Structure of riboflavin.

Bacteria are susceptible to riboflavin-mediated photoinactivation. Treatment of pooled platelet components suspended in 10% synthetic media, 90% carryover plasma, with 50 μM riboflavin and 6 J/cm^2 UVA light, resulted in inactivation of an average of 5.1 log *S. epidermidis*, 4.7 log *E. coli*, 4.5 log *Staphylococcus aureus*, 3.1 log *Bacillus cereus*, and 5.5 log *Klebsiella pneumoniae*.[45] No information is available about whether the lower level of inactivation observed with *B. cereus* was due to a possible resistance of spores to riboflavin photoinactivation. In another study, investigators utilized 20 μM riboflavin and 419 nm visible light (80 J/cm^2/minute) for 23 minutes to inactivate six bacterial strains in 80% platelet storage solution:20% Mueller-Hinton broth.[46] The solution was inoculated with three strains of coagulase-negative *Staphylococcus* species, one strain of *S. aureus*, and one strain of *Pseudomonas aeruginosa* at log or stationary phase growth to produce a final bacterial count of 100 colony-forming units (CFU)/mL. Inoculated samples were divided into controls and riboflavin-phototreated groups and stored with agitation at room temperature for 7 days. None of the riboflavin-treated samples resulted in bacterial growth after 7-day storage; all control samples revealed growth that reached 10^8 CFU/mL within 24 hours.

The in-vitro properties of riboflavin-phototreated platelets were investigated under conditions that documented >5.85 log of the model virus, bovine viral diarrhea virus.[47] Ten units of platelets were suspended in 27% plasma, 73% synthetic storage media, and 50 μM riboflavin. The units were subsequently illuminated with 5 J/cm^2 of 419 nm visible light. A number of platelet in-vitro properties were measured during 5-day room temperature storage and compared to 21 untreated control units stored in plasma. At the conclusion of 5 days of storage, there was no significant change in pH, pO_2, lactate levels/1000 cells, cell count, heat shock recovery response, or qualitative ability to swirl of riboflavin-treated units compared with unpaired untreated controls. Riboflavin phototreatment did cause a twofold increase in GMP-140 expression ($p<0.05$), indicative of platelet activation.

Another investigation focused on in-vivo survival and recovery of riboflavin-phototreated platelets.[48] In a primate platelet survival study, investigators suspended cynomolgus macaque platelets in 27% plasma, 73% synthetic storage media. The concentration of riboflavin was not given but is presumed to be 50 μM. Radiolabeled riboflavin-containing platelets were illuminated with 10 J/cm^2 419 nm visible light. Untreated control platelets were suspended in plasma, radiolabeled, and infused. Treated and control platelets had somewhat similar survival curves, with estimated half-life values of 33 and 38 hours, respectively. Although the conditions of macaque platelet survival experiments differed from those utilized for bacterial inactivation in plasma concentration, light dose, and light source, the use of less concentrated plasma levels would appear to represent more stringent conditions if the same light source and dose were utilized in the two studies. Nevertheless, additional studies conducted under the same conditions are warranted. In addition to these validations, it would be important to demonstrate the hemostatic potential of riboflavin-treated platelets.

Unlike many of the other agents utilized for pathogen reduction, riboflavin is a vitamin and, as such, is less likely to produce toxic effects in recipients. However, riboflavin is converted to lumichrome when illuminated under physiologic conditions.[49] Investigators have found no evidence of cytotoxicity after incubating L929 mouse fibroblasts with up to 90 μM lumichrome. Intravenous administration of 900 μg/kg of lumichrome in 0.9% saline into mice resulted in no observable acute toxicity. Finally, exposure of up to 21.8 μg/mL (90 μM) lumicrome to Ames tester strains resulted in no evidence of mutagenicity in either the presence or absence of S9 metabolic activating fraction.

S-59 (Amotosalen) and Ultraviolet A Light

The psoralen, S-59, has been synthesized for photoinactivation of pathogens in platelet components (Fig 9-4).[50] Psoralens intercalate between nucleic acid bases. Upon illumination with UVA light, psoralens produce monoadducts and diadducts with pyrimidine bases in nucleic acids. These monoadducts and diadducts, or crosslinks, prevent polymerase passage across the lesions and thus prevent pathogen replication.

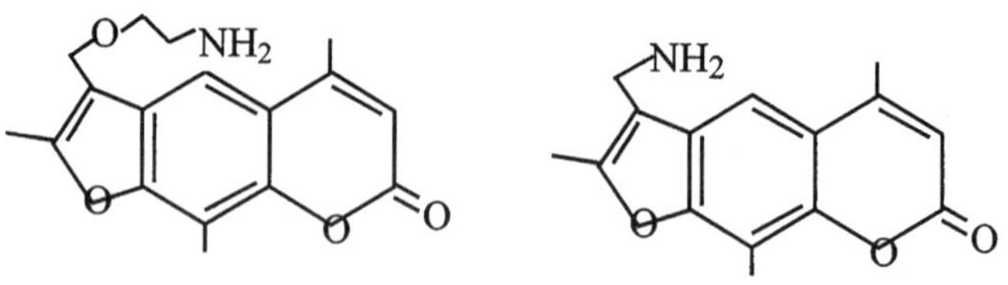

NH_2 O O O O

NH_2 O O O

Figure 9-4. Structure of S-59 (left) and 4′-aminomethyl-4,5′,8-trimethylpsoralen (right).

Investigators have generally utilized 150 μM S-59 in platelets suspended in 30% plasma and 70% synthetic medium, with UVA light exposures of 3 J/cm^2. Under these conditions, >6.6 log *S. epidermidis*, >5.6 log of *K. pneumoniae*, >6.9 log of *Lactobacillus*, >6.5 log of *Bifidabacterium adolescentis*, >6.7 log of *Propionibacterium acnes*, and > 7.0 log of *Clostridium perfringens* were inactivated in apheresis platelets.[51,52] In another series of experiments utilizing pools of buffy-coat-derived platelets and identical photoinactivation conditions, S-59 treatment completely inactivated *S. epidermidis*, *S. aureus*, *Enterococcus faecalis*, *Enterobacter aerogenes*, *P. aeruginosa*, and *Serratia marcescens* with initial inoculi of 3900, 340, 260, 670, 520, and 950 CFU/mL, respectively.[53] None of these bacterial species could be cultured from treated units stored for 7 days at room temperature but could be readily cultured from untreated controls. S-59 and light treatment failed to produce culture-negative platelets in one experiment with 12 CFU/mL of *B. cereus* but yielded culture-negative platelets in another experiment with 180 CFU/mL. The authors attributed the inconsistent inactivation of *B. cereus* to the presence of bacterial spores, which may be insensitive to photoinactivation.

Two studies have demonstrated that *T. cruzi* trypomastigotes are sensitive to psoralen and light-mediated inactivation. In the first study, 170 μM of the psoralen, 4′-aminomethyl-4,5′,8-trimethylpsoralen (AMT), was utilized with 4.2 J/cm^2 UVA light in platelet concentrates containing 0.35 mM of the antioxidant, rutin.[54] Using a step to enrich for mobile trypomastigotes involving centrifuging phototreated and control units and incubating 1 to 2 hours to allow mobile trypomastigotes to exit the pellet, a dilution series of supernatant was incubated with LLC-MK2 cells and subsequently assayed for infection microscopically for the presence or absence of trypomastigote forms. Phototreatment resulted in >4.5 log inactivation of *T. cruzi*. AMT and UVA treatment had much less impact on short-term inhibition of trypomastigote motility. At 2 hours after AMT and 4.2 J/cm^2 UVA light treatment, the fraction of mobile trypomastigotes was only reduced by approximately 0.25 log, demonstrating that the pellet enrichment step had little impact on subsequent trypomastigote viability measurements. In a second study, the psoralen S-59 and UVA light were used to inactivate *T. cruzi* in platelet concentrates.[55] Infectivity was measured by serial dilution of control and phototreated samples, infection of 3T3 cells, and subsequent microscopic evaluation. Using 150 μM S-59 and 3 J/cm^2 UVA light, >5.4 log inactivation of trypomastigotes was documented.

In another study, the psoralen AMT was utilized to study the inactivation of the obligate intracellular bacterium, *Orientia tsutsugamushi*, which is also known as the scrub typhus organism.[56] Platelet concentrates were deliberately inoculated with infected mononuclear cells and subsequently treated with 0.86 to 138 μM AMT and 5 J/cm^2 UVA light. The investigators used a variety of assays for the detection of *O. tsutsugamushi*, including indirect fluorescence antibody, direct fluorescence antibody, Giemsa staining, an in-vitro PCR assay, and a mouse infectivity assay. Intracranial infusion of mice with 1.9×10^4 to 2.0×10^5 organisms resulted in the death of all mice 12 to 17 days after infection; all mice receiving phototreated platelets containing initial AMT concentrations of AMT 0.86 μM or more lived for more than 2 weeks with no signs of infection as determined by examination of blood samples using direct or indirect fluorescence antibody, Giemsa staining, or PCR. However, all mice receiving control platelets showed evidence of infection by these assays. Based on the published information, it is not possible to calculate the extent of AMT photoinactivation of *O. tsutsugamushi* in these experiments.

The susceptibility of *Plasmodium falciparum* intraerythrocytic form and *Leishmania mexicana* metacyclic promastigotes to S-59 photoinactivation was investigated in another series of studies.[57] Apheresis platelets were deliberately inoculated with approximately 10^6 infectious organisms, suspended in 35% plasma and 65% synthetic medium, and treated with 150 μM of S-59 and 1, 2, or 3 J/cm^2 UVA light. Treated and control samples were titrated by unspecified in-vitro culture techniques. Using as little as 1 J/cm^2 UVA light exposure with S-59, >7.0 log *P. falciparum* and >5.2 log *L. mexicana* were inactivated.

Under the described pathogen reduction conditions, treatment with S-59 and UVA light results in the retention of most in-vitro platelet properties.[51] No change was noted between treated and control units for pH, pCO_2, HCO_3^-, platelet morphology, platelet count, plasma glucose, lactose, percentage of aggregation, secretory ATP, platelet shape change, and hypotonic shock response after 5 days of room temperature storage. Platelets treated with S-59 and UVA light have 13% greater levels of P-selectin and 20% greater levels pO_2 than untreated controls. The posttransfusional autologous recovery and survival of treated and control rhesus monkey platelets were comparable.[51] Using crossed immunoelectrophoresis and flow cytometry assays, no evidence for the production of neoantigens by S-59 phototreatment was observed.[51]

Several clinical trials have been performed using S-59 and UVA-light-treated platelets. In an early study using healthy human subjects, treated platelets were stored for 5 days, radiolabeled, and autologously infused.[58] Treated platelets had 15.5% reduced survival and 20.9% reduced life span compared with untreated stored platelets ($p<0.05$). However, actual values of survival and life span for treated platelets were within the low range of published values for untreated platelets. In a second clinical trial, the ability of S-59-treated platelets to reduce the bleeding time in thrombocytopenic patients was investigated.[59] Infusion of either treated or control platelets resulted in comparable reduction (ranging from 38 to 71%) of the bleeding times relative to the bleeding times of 13 patients measured just before transfusion. In the same study, analysis of five additional patients receiving treated and control platelets revealed that patients receiving S-59 and UVA light-treated platelets had a 31.5% reduction of 1-hour corrected count increment and a 29.5% reduction of 24-hour corrected count increment relative to untreated platelets.

In a third clinical trial, the safety and efficacy of S-59 phototreatment were investigated in a 100-patient, two-arm study in Europe.[60,61] Control and photochemically treated arms had similar numbers of patients experience transfusion reactions or suffer from major hemorrhage. Patients receiving photochemically treated platelets required, on average, 33.9% more transfusions than patients receiving control platelets and had 9.3% fewer platelets per unit than untreated platelets. The average total number of platelets utilized by patients in the photochemically treated and control arms were similar. Similar to the results obtained in the previous clinical study, the 24-hour corrected count increment measured in patients receiving photochemically treated platelets was 31% less than that measured from patients receiving control platelets. However, the 1-hour corrected count increment was similar in both treated and control arms. Finally, there was no difference in the hemostatic effectiveness, as measured by Grade 2 or greater bleeding, of photochemically treated platelets compared with control platelets in a large study of 645 thrombocytopenic patients conducted in the United States.[62] However, 1-hour posttransfusion platelet counts in the treated arm were 10,000/µL less than those measured in the control group after adjusting for platelet dose and pretransfusion platelet counts. In addition, the mean number of prophylactic platelet transfusions per patient increased 41% in the photochemically treated group compared with the control group ($p<0.05$). Prophylactic platelet transfusions were triggered by platelet counts below 10,000 or 20,000/µL. For actively bleeding patients, no difference was observed in the mean number of therapeutic platelet transfusions per patient between treated and control arms.

Results from a number of genotoxicity assays have been published for S-59.[63] S-59 is positive in the Ames bacterial mutagenicity test. Using the *Salmonella* tester strain, TA1537, S-59 was positive at 44 and 103 µg/mL when samples were incubated in the presence or absence of S9 microsomal fraction for metabolic activation, respectively. S-59 was negative at concentrations ≤65 µg/mL in the mouse lymphoma assay performed in the presence of metabolic activation, but positive in the assay at concentrations >7.5 μg/mL in the absence of metabolic activation. In the chromosomal abberation assay, S-59 was positive at concentrations ≥5 μg/mL in the absence of metabolic activation and also positive at 46 μg/mL in the presence of metabolic activation. S-59 was negative in an in-vivo unscheduled DNA synthesis assay at doses as high as 34 mg/kg and negative in an in-vivo mouse micronucleus assay at doses as high as 66 mg/kg.

A fraction of S-59 is converted to photoproducts following UVA illumination. After UVA illumination of S-59-treated platelets, there was no evidence of genotoxicity of 2 to 2.5 μg/mL residual S-59 and 8 to 10 μg/mL of photoproducts when the chromosomal aberration assay was performed.[63] Under similar UVA light treatment conditions, S-59-phototreated platelets were negative in the Ames test and in the mouse lymphoma assay.[63] The investigators have included an affinity removal device to reduce the concentration of free S-59. The use of this device should decrease the risk of genotoxicity for recipients of phototreated product.

A heterologous transgenic p53 mouse model was utilized to investigate the carcinogenic potential of platelets or plasma phototreated with S-59.[64] Mice were treated three-times a week with control and phototreated components for 26 weeks. The dose range was the expected 26-week aggregate clinical exposure (1 mg/kg) of S-59 treated platelets (with use of an S-59 removal device) to 1000 clinical exposures. At the end of the study, there was no evidence of carcinogenicity in mice receiving S-59-treated product. No results from photocarcinogenicity studies have been reported.

Conclusions

Pathogen reduction systems for cellular blood components offer the promise to reduce the residual risk of infection from tested pathogens, diminish the current risk from untested pathogens, and lessen the future risk from unknown pathogens. The efficacy of risk reduction from unknown agents cannot be ascertained. In addition, not all infectious agents are susceptible to complete inactivation, either because some infectious agents have unusually high bioburdens or because the structures of some infectious agents are impermeable to the inactivating compound.

All of the inactivation methods described in this chapter target nucleic acid. As a result, considerable care must be exercised to evaluate the potential for genotoxic risk to transfusion recipients. In addition, thought must be given to the potential risk to blood bank workers in case of accidental exposure. Because accidents during the inactivation process could potentially expose workers to high concentrations of active agents before their breakdown, conversion to photoproducts, and/or removal, genotoxic risks to staff during an accident may be greater than genotoxic risks to transfusion recipients.

Although all of the described agents target nucleic acid, there is still some collateral damage to red cells or platelets. In many cases, this has been documented by changes in red cell or platelet in-vitro properties, decreases in recovery or survival, changes in corrected count increment, or increased utilization of components in patients receiving units that have been subjected to inactivation methods.

How does one weigh the risk of infectious disease from currently tested blood to the risk from pathogen reduction methods, which might include new toxicity risks, changes in blood component storage properties, and/or decreases in blood cell recovery or survival? For countries that routinely perform HIV and HCV antibody tests and NAT, as well as test for HBV, HTLV, and screen for syphilis, the current infectious disease risk is low and would be expected to further decline with the implementation of bacterial screening and West Nile virus NAT. It is possible that standard toxicity assays may not be adequate to predict whether the chance of serious toxicities are less than the current chance of fatal virus, bacteria, or parasite infection. In addition, experience from clinical trials involving fewer than 800 individuals is inadequate for the prediction of very low-frequency adverse events. Therefore, surveillance efforts during implementation will be required in order to determine whether the frequency of serious adverse events of a pathogen reduction process is less than the current risk of infectious disease transmission by transfusion.

References

1. Schreiber GB, Busch MP, Kleinman SH, Korelitz JJ. The risk of transfusion-transmitted viral infections. N Engl J Med 1996;334:1685-9.
2. National Heart, Lung, and Blood Institute. In vitro inactivation of viruses in blood components. RFA HL-00-010. January 18, 2000. [Available at http://grants.nih.gov/grants/guide/rfa-files/RFA-HL-00- 010.html].
3. Dodd RY. Germs, gels, and genomes: A personal recollection of 30 years in blood safety testing. In: Stramer S, ed. Blood safety in the new millennium. Bethesda, MD: American Association of Blood Banks, 2000:97-122.
4. Lee J. FDA surveillance for bacterial safety of blood. Presented at the FDA/CBER Bacterial Contamination of Platelets Workshop, Bethesda, MD, September 24, 1999.
5. Ness P, Braine H, King K, et al. Single-donor platelets reduce the risk of septic platelet transfusion reactions. Transfusion 2001;41:857-61.
6. Kuehnert MJ, Roth VR, Haley NR, et al. Transfusion-transmitted bacterial infection in the United States, 1998 through 2000. Transfusion 2001;41(12):1493-9.
7. Dobroszycki J, Herwaldt BL, Boctor F, et al. A cluster of transfusion-associated babesiosis cases traced to a single asymptomatic donor. JAMA 1999;281(10):927-30.
8. Herwaldt BL, Neitzel DF, Gorlin JB, et al. Transmission of *Babesia microti* in Minnesota through four blood donations from the same donor over a 6-month period. Transfusion 2002;42:1154-8.
9. Kjemtrup AM, Lee B, Fritz CL, et al. Investigation of transfusion transmission of a WA1-type babesial parasite to a premature infant in California. Transfusion 2002;42:1482-7.
10. Cimo PL, Luper WE, Scouros MA. Transfusion-associated Chagas' disease in Texas: Report of a case. Tex Med 1993;89:48-50.
11. Leiby DA, Lenes BA, Tibbals MA, Tames-Olmedo MT. Prospective evaluation of a patient with *Trypanosoma cruzi* infection transmitted by transfusion. N Engl J Med 1999;341:1237-9.
12. Cook D, Wollowitz D. Method for inactivating pathogens in red cell compositions using quinacrine mustard. US Patent #5691132, 1997.

13. Greenman WM, Grass JA, Talib S, et al. Method of treating leukocytes, leukocyte compositions and methods of use thereof. European Patent Application WO 99/03976, 1998.
14. Stassinopoulos A, Mababangloob RS, Dupuis KW, Johnson KM. Bacterial inactivation in leukoreduced PRBC treated with Helinx™ (abstract). Transfusion 2000;40(Suppl):38S.
15. Cook D, Stassinopoulos A, Merritt J, et al. Inactivation of pathogens in packed red blood cells (PRBC) concentrates using S-303 (abstract). Blood 1997;90(Suppl):409a.
16. Cook D, Stassinopoulos A. Methods for quenching pathogen inactivators in biological materials. US Patent #6,270,952, 2001.
17. Cook D, Stassinopoulos A, Wollowitz S, et al. In vivo analysis of packed red blood cells treated with S-303 to inactivate pathogens (abstract). Blood 1998;92(Suppl 1):503a.
18. Hambleton J, Greenwalt T, Viele M, et al. Post transfusion recovery after multiple exposures to red blood cell concentrates (RBCS) treated with a novel pathogen inactivation (P.I.) process (abstract). Blood 1999;94(Suppl 1):376a.
19. Rogers AM, Back KC. Comparative mutagenicity of 4 DNA-intercalating agents in L5178Y mouse lymphoma cells. Mutat Res 1982;102:447-55.
20. Haglund U, Zech L. Simultaneous staining of sister chromatid exchanges and Q-bands in human chromosomes after treatment with methyl methane sulphonate, quinacrine mustard and quinacrine. Hum Genet 1979;49:307-17.
21. Ciaravino V, Stassinopoulos A, Singh Y, McCullough T. Intercept red blood cells are not genotoxic or carcinogenic in a series of in vitro and in vivo tests (abstract). Blood 2002;100(Suppl):143b.
22. Budowsky EL, Ackerman SK, Purmal AA, et al. Methods and compositions for the selective modification of nucleic acids. US Patent #6,093,564, 2000.
23. Bahnemann HG. Inactivation of viruses in serum with binary ethyleneimine. J Clin Microbiol 1976;3:209-10.
24. Hulskotte EG, Ding ME, Norley SG, et al. Chemical inactivation of recombinant vaccinia viruses and the effects on antigenicity and immunogenicity of recombinant simian immunodeficiency virus envelope glycoproteins. Vaccine 1997;15:1839-45.
25. Yamada H, Imoto T, Noshita S. Modification of catalytic groups in lysozyme with ethylenimine. Biochemistry 1982;21:2187-92.
26. Okazaki K, Yamada H, Imoto T. A convenient S-2-aminoethylation of cysteinyl residues in reduced proteins. Anal Biochem 1985;149:516-20.
27. Zavizion B, Serebryanik D, Serebryanik I, et al. Prevention of *Yersinia enterocolitica*, *Pseudomonas fluorescens*, and *Pseudomonas putida* outgrowth in deliberately inoculated blood by a novel pathogen-reduction process. Transfusion 2003;43:135-42.
28. Zavizion B, Serebryanik D, Purmal A. Collection system equivalency using the INACTINE™ process for pathogen inactivation: Bacterial inactivation assessment (abstract). Transfusion 2001;41(Suppl):89S.

29. Pereira M, Serebryanik D, Purmal A. Inactivation of virulent *Trypanosoma cruzi* trypomastigotes by the INACTINE™ process (abstract). Transfusion 2001;41(Suppl):87S.
30. Zavizion B, Mather T, Miller N. INACTINE PEN110 chemistry eradicates the parasite that causes babesiosis (abstract). Transfusion 2002; 42(Suppl):93S.
31. AuBuchon JP, Pickard CA, Herschel LH, et al. Production of pathogen-inactivated RBC concentrates using PEN110 chemistry: A Phase I clinical study. Transfusion 2002;42:146-52.
32. Mintz P, Snyder E, Burks S, et al. Pathogen inactivated red blood cells using INACTINE™ technology demonstrate 24 hour post transfusion recovery equal to untreated red cells after 42 days of storage (abstract). Blood 2001;98(Suppl 1):709a-10a.
33. Valencia R, Mason JM, Woodruff RC, et al. Chemical mutagenesis testing in *Drosophila*. III. Results of 48 coded compounds tested for the National Toxicology Program. Environ Mutagen 1985;7:325-48.
34. Nishi Y, Hasegawa MM, Taketomi M, et al. Comparison of 6-thioguanine-resistant mutation and sister chromatid exchanges in Chinese hamster V79 cells with forty chemical and physical agents. Cancer Res 1984;44:3270-9.
35. Siboulet R, Grinfeld S, Deparis P, et al. Micronuclei in red blood cells of the newt Pleurodeles waltl Michah: Induction with X-rays and chemicals. Mutat Res 1984;125:275-81.
36. Chapman J, Keys D. Lack of toxicity of PEN110 treated red blood cells without PEN110 removal in New Zealand white rabbits (abstract). Transfusion 2001;41(Suppl):89S.
37. Chapman J, Moore K. High exposure to the pathogen inactivation compound PEN110 does not effect fertility or embryonic development in rats (abstract). Transfusion 2002;42(Suppl):17S.
38. Joshi PC. Comparison of the DNA-damaging property of photosensitised riboflavin via singlet oxygen ($^1O_2$) and superoxide radical O_2^-. mechanisms. Toxicol Lett 1985;26:211-17.
39. Ito K, Inoue S, Yamamoto K, Kawanishi S. 8-hydroxyguanosine formation at the 5′ site of 5′-GG-3′ sequences in double-stranded DNA by UV radiation with riboflavin. J Biol Chem 1993;268:13221-7.
40. Ennever JF, Speck WT. Short communication. Photochemical reactions of riboflavin: Covalent binding to DNA and to poly (dA) . poly (dT). Pediatr Res 1983;17:234-6.
41. Ali N, Upreti RK, Srivastava LP, et al. Membrane damaging potential of photosensitized riboflavin. Indian J Exp Biol 1991;29:818-22.
42. Ghazy FS, Kimura T, Muranishi S. The photodynamic action of riboflavin on erythrocytes. Life Sciences 1977;21:1703-8.
43. Tapia G, Silva E. Photo-induced riboflavin binding to the tryptophan residues of bovine and human serum albumins. Radiat Environ Biophys 1991;30:131-8.
44. Diaz M, Becker MI, De Ioannes AE, Silva E. Development of monoclonal antibodies against a riboflavin-tryptophan photoinduced

adduct: Reactivity to eye lens proteins. Photochem Photobiol 1996;63: 762-7.

45. Goodrich L, Douglas I, Urioste M. Riboflavin photoinactivation procedure inactivates significant levels of bacteria and produces a culture negative product (abstract). Transfusion 2002;42(Suppl):16S.
46. Palavecino EL, Jacobs MR, Goodrich RP, et al. Photochemical decontamination of bacteria: Analysis of log and stationary growth phases (abstract). Transfusion 2001;42(Suppl):88S-9S.
47. Goodrich LL, Hasen ET, Gampp D, et al. Riboflavin pathogen inactivation process yields good platelet cell quality and expedient viral kill (abstract). Blood 2001;98(Suppl):540a.
48. Goodrich RP, Woolum M, Hasen E, Zavorskas P. Recovery and survival kinetics of radiolabelled platelets following treatment with a riboflavin based pathogen inactivation procedure (abstract). Blood 2001;98(Suppl):541a.
49. Piper JT, Murphy SE, Schuyler R, et al. Evaluation of acute toxicity and genotoxicity risks associated with the riboflavin photoproduct lumichrome (abstract). Transfusion 2001;41(Suppl):90S.
50. Wollowitz S. Fundamentals of the psoralen-based Helinx™ technology for inactivation of infectious pathogens and leukocytes in platelets and plasma. Semin Hematol 2001;38(Suppl 11):4-11.
51. Lin L, Cook DN, Wisehahn GP, et al. Photochemical inactivation of viruses and bacteria in platelet concentrates by use of a novel psoralen and long-wavelength ultraviolet light. Transfusion 1997;37:423-35.
52. Savoor AR, Mababangloob R, Kinsey J, et al. The intercept blood system for platelets inactivates anaerobic bacteria (abstract). Transfusion 2002;42(Suppl):92S.
53. Knutson F, Alfonso R, Dupuis K, et al. Photochemical inactivation of bacteria and HIV in buffy-coat-derived platelet concentrates under conditions that preserve in vitro platelet function. Vox Sang 2000;78:209-16.
54. Gottlieb P, Margolis-Nunno H, Robinson R, et al. Inactivation of *Trypanosoma cruzi* trypomastigote forms in blood components with a psoralen and ultraviolet A light. Photochem Photobiol 1996;63:562-5.
55. Van Voorhis WC, Barrett LK, Eastman RT, et al. *Trypanosoma cruzi* inactivation in human platelet concentrates and plasma by a psoralen (Amotosalen HCl) and long-wavelength UV. Antimicrob Agents Chemo 2003;47:475-9.
56. Belanger KJ, Kelly DJ, Mettille FC, et al. Psoralen photochemical inactivation of *Orientia tsutsugamushi* in platelet concentrates. Transfusion 2000;40;1503-7.
57. Van Voorhis W, Alfonso R, Barrett L, et al. Intercept blood system for platelets, using Helinx® technology, inactivates the protozoa of malaria, Chagas' disease and Leishmaniasis (abstract). Blood 2002; 100(Suppl):708a.
58. Corash L, Behrman B, Rheinschmidt M, et al. Post-transfusion viability and tolerability of photochemically treated platelet concentrates (abstract). Blood 1997;90(Suppl 1):267a.

59. Slichter SJ, Corash L, Grabowski M, et al. Viability and hemostatic function of photochemically treated (PCT) platelets (PLTS) in thrombocytopenic patients (abstract). Blood 1999;94(Suppl 1):376a.
60. Van Rhenen D, Gulliksson H, Pamphilon D, et al. S-59 (HELINX) photochemically treated platelets (ptls) are safe and effective for support of thrombocytopenia: Results of the EUROSPRITE phase 3 trial (abstract). Blood 2000;96(Suppl 1):819a.
61. Van Rhenen D, Gulliksson H, Cazenave J-P, et al. Transfusion of pooled buffy coat platelet components prepared with photochemical pathogen inactivation treatment: The euroSPRITE trial. Blood 2003; 101:2426-33.
62. Slichter SJ, Murphy S, Buchholz D, et al. INTERCEPT platelets (plts) and conventional plts provide comparable hemostatic responses in thrombocytopenic patients (pts): The SPRINT trial (abstract). Blood 2002;100(Suppl 2):141b.
63. Ciaravino V. Preclinical safety of a nucleic acid-targeted Helinx™ compound: A clinical perspective. Semin Hematol 2001;38(Suppl 11): 12-19.
64. Ciaravino V, Sullivan T, McCullough T. Intercept-treated platelets and plasma are not carcinogenic in a sensitive transgenic p53 mouse model (abstract). Vox Sang 2002;83(Suppl 2):110.

Appendix 1. Association Bulletin #02-8

ASSOCIATION BULLETIN

#02-8

Date: December 10, 2002

To: AABB Members

From: Roger Dodd, PhD - President
Karen Shoos Lipton, JD - Chief Executive Officer

Re: Update on Bacterial Contamination of Platelet Units

This Association Bulletin updates AB 96-06 and provides members with additional information regarding the frequency, cause, outcomes, prevention, and detection of bacterial contamination of platelet units. This bulletin does not establish new AABB policy with regard to this long-recognized problem, but is intended to apprise members of new information about, and additional means of dealing with, this important transfusion risk. In addition, the Standards Committee, with input and support from the Transfusion Transmitted Diseases and Clinical Transfusion Medicine Committees, has developed draft standards for incorporation into *Standards for Blood Banks and Transfusion Services, 22nd Edition.* A proposed new standard, 5.1.5.1, incorporates a requirement that facilities have "method(s) to detect bacterial contamination in all platelet components." Standard 5.6.2 has been revised to require that skin at the venipuncture site be prepared with tincture of iodine, while permitting the use of chlorhexidine for donors who are allergic or sensitive to iodine. The proposed standards, which are available for comment until January 8, 2003, are based, in part, on data contained in the attached references. These references are provided for your consideration in preparing comments on the proposed draft standards and in addressing the risk of bacterial contamination of platelet units.

Bacterial contamination has been recognized for decades as being a significant risk associated with the room-temperature storage of platelets. As other infectious risks of transfusion have been reduced, the magnitude and relative importance of bacterial contamination of platelets has become more apparent. The need to address and interdict this problem is clear. Although various innovative strategies have been and are being developed to address this risk, none appears to provide a perfect solution; thus, it may be appropriate to consider multiple approaches to reduce the greatest infectious risk faced by recipients of platelet transfusions.

In considering transfusion risks and their amelioration, the AABB Clinical Transfusion Medicine Committee requested that Mark Brecher, MD, University of North Carolina, Chapel Hill, NC, prepare an annotated bibliography of the key scientific literature pertaining to bacterial contamination of platelets. This document is included in this association bulletin to provide authoritative information to members regarding the scope and importance of the problem of bacterial contamination of blood components. Members are encouraged to review this bibliography as they seek additional ways to reduce significant transfusion risks.

Members are urged to begin to consider how their practices of blood banking and transfusion medicine may be modified to reduce the risk of collecting or transfusing a bacterially contaminated unit. The problems posed by a bacterial inoculum -- including initially low concentrations, but potentially rapid growth later in storage -- are different from the viral threats that recently have received attention and may call for novel approaches. While further informatior and recommendations are being developed by the association on these issues, the following measures are mentioned for consideration as potentially useful and applicable:

Prevention or Limitation of Contamination

- Use of an alcohol/tincture of iodine skin preparation method appears to be associated with reduced contamination.

- When approved by FDA and marketed, blood collection sets that allow diversion of the first volume of blood away from the collection set may prevent skin contaminants from inoculating the unit.

- Limiting the storage period of platelets limits the time period during which contaminating bacteria may multiply to dangerous levels; however, with an already limited storage period for this component, the supply ramifications of this approach need to be balanced against its potential benefits.

Detection of Contamination

- Observation of loss of "swirling" in platelet limits may be a clue that they are bacterially contaminated. Platelets lose their discoid form and their ability to align under flow conditions when the pH falls below 6.2, as may occur because of bacterial production of organic acids. However, the sensitivity of this technique is uncertain, and challenges of training as well as concerns with reproducibility and documentation of results need to be addressed. In addition, platelets may lose their discoid form for reasons unrelated to bacterial contamination.

- Alterations in biochemical measurements that can be affected by bacterial growth, such as pH and glucose concentration, may indicate bacterial contamination. These analytes may be measured by instruments or through use of reagent dipsticks. In general, however, bacterial concentrations are likely to exceed clinically significant levels before these analytes become significantly abnormal.

- An aliquot of a platelet unit may be examined microscopically by Gram or Wright's stain or a fluorescent stain (eg, acridine orange) to detect bacteria that may be present. The sensitivity of these techniques is approximately that of or slightly better than the sensitivity of biochemical analyses. A variable number of false-positive identifications do occur.

- Culture of an aliquot of a unit may be used to directly detect the presence of bacteria. The volume cultured and the time between donation and culturing combine to determine the sensitivity of the technique. Two commercially available techniques that depend on bacterial growth for their detection have been approved by the FDA as quality control systems for platelet sterility; one technique identifies growth through the carbon dioxide generated by bacterial growth, while the other detects growth through consumption of oxygen by the organisms.

Members are encouraged to review the attached information carefully and consider how the risk of bacterial contamination of platelet units can be addressed in their facilities.

Annotated Bibliography: Bacterial Contamination of Platelets

Prepared for the Clinical Transfusion Medicine Committee by
Mark Brecher, MD
University of North Carolina

Note: The inclusion and discussion of an article in this listing does not imply endorsement of the technique by the AABB.

Incidence

Chiu EKW, Yuen KY, Lie AKW, Liang R, Lau YL, Lee ACW, Kwong YL, Wong S, Ng MH, Chan TK. A prospective study of symptomatic bacteremia following platelet transfusion and of its management. Transfusion 1994; 34:950-54.

> In a study of symptomatic bacteremia following platelet transfusion in 161 bone marrow transplant recipients in Hong Kong, it was found that 1 in 2,000 units of platelet concentrates were bacterially contaminated. This translated to 1 in 350 pooled platelets being contaminated. Of those patients who were febrile (elevation of temperature of $\geq$ 1°C) following platelet transfusion, 1 in 4 (27%) were found to have received a bacterially contaminated unit. Of those found to have a $\geq$ 2°C rise in temperature following a platelet transfusion, 50% were found to have received a bacterially contaminated unit. In this multiply transfused patient population, the chance of receiving a bacterially contaminated platelet was 1 in 16. Of the 10 patients known to have received a bacterially contaminated unit, 4 suffered from septic shock.

Yomtovian R, Lazarus HM, Goodnough LT, et al. A prospective microbiologic surveillance program to detect and prevent the transfusion of bacterially contaminated platelets. Transfusion 1993;33:902-09.

> Aerobic solid media cultures (incubated for 48 hours) of 3,141 unit random donor pools (prepared from14,481 units) and 2,476 single donor pools were prospectively cultured. Six pools (1of 524 random donor pools or 0.19% or 1:2,414 source units) were contaminated and none of the single donor apheresis bags were contaminated. In 3 of 4 patients who received contaminated platelets, no signs or symptoms were manifest. In platelets aged one to five days, the sensitivity and specificity of a Gram stain was 80% and 99.96% respectively. In four-to five-day-old platelets, the sensitivity was increased to 100%, with a specificity of 99.93%. The true-positive results were associated with bacterial concentrations >10^6 CFU/mL.

Sazama K. Bacteria in blood for transfusion. A review. Arch Pathol Lab Med 1994;118:350-365.

> Of 52 reported cases of bacterial contamination of platelets culled from world literature, 10 were associated with death (19.6% or approximately 1 in 5).

Morrow JF, Braine HG, Kickler TS, Ness PM, Dick JK, Fuller AK. Septic reactions to platelet transfusions. A persistent problem. JAMA 1991:266:555-8.

This paper reports 6 cases (1:1,700 incidence) of transfusion-associated sepsis in recipients of pooled random donor platelets. Only 1 of 20,000 apheresis units was associated with transfusion-associated sepsis. Platelets stored for 5 days were associated with clinical signs and symptoms 5 times more frequently than those stored for 4 days or less.

Perez P, Salmi R, Follea G, et al. Determinants of transfusion associated bacterial contamination results of the French Bacthem case-control study. Transfusion 2001;41:862-72.

Summary of data from France over a 2-year period (1997-1998) of transfusion-associated bacterial contamination. Of 16 cases of bacterial contamination associated with platelet transfusion 9 (56%) resulted in severe sepsis or shock. Estimates of incidence of life-threatening reactions was 9.4 per million (1:106,000) units for single unit random-donor platelet concentrates and 17.7 per million (1:56,500) for apheresis platelet concentrates.

Kuehnert MJ, Roth VR, Haley NR, et al. Transfusion-transmitted bacterial infection in the United States, 1998 through 2000. Transfusion 2001;41:1493-99.

A 2 year prospective passive reporting system of transfusion-transmitted sepsis in the United States. Twenty-nine cases of bacterial contaminated platelets met very strict clinical case criteria (e.g., reactions occurring within 4 hours of transfusion), 6 cases resulted in death (21%).

Serious Hazards of Transfusion (SHOT) report for 1999-2000 and for 2000-2001. (cumulative data 01/10/1995-30/09/2002) http://www.shot.demon.co.uk/toc.htm.

Summary of the Serious Hazards of Transfusion Study from the United Kingdom. From 1995 to 2002, 17 cases of platelet-associated transfusion-transmitted bacterial infection were reported. Death was attributed to the infection in 5 of the 17 cases (29%).

Random versus Single Donor apheresis

Ness PM, Braine HG, King K, et al. Single donor platelets reduce the risk of septic transfusion reactions. Transfusion 2001;41:857-61.

This paper summarized the clinical experience from Johns Hopkins from the years 1986 to 1998. During this period the hospital moved from transfusing 48.3% random platelet pools and 51.7 % single donor apheresis platelets to 99.4% single donor apheresis platelets. The incidence of clinical septic events related to platelets went from 1:4,818 to 1:15,098. The risk was 5.4-fold higher with random pooled platelets than with single donor apheresis platelets. The overall clinical sepsis rate was approximately 1:2,500 for random donor pools and 1:13,400 single donor apheresis transfusions, and the related mortality was approximately 1:17,000 for random donor pools and 1:61,000 for single donor apheresis platelets. This paper concluded that the use of single donor apheresis platelets is a simple means of reducing septic platelet transfusion reactions.

Presentation of reactions

Rhame FS, Root RK, MacLowry JD, Dadisman TA, Bennett JV. *Salmonella septicemia* from platelet transfusions. Study of an outbreak traced to a hematogenous carrier *of Salmonella cholerae-suis.* Ann Intern Med. 1973;78:633-41.

> This was an epidemiologic investigation of an outbreak of *Salmonella choleraseus* sepsis in 7 patients at the NIH Clinical Center that was traced to one repeat platelet donor subsequently found to have an occult chronic osteomyelitis. The time to the onset of illness ranged from 5 to12 days (mean 8.6 days). One patient died, and two had long-term recurrences. This paper illustrates the long delay that can result between platelet transfusion and the onset of clinical symptoms, leading to under diagnosis of post- transfusion sepsis.

Roth VR, Arduino MJ, Nobiletti J, et al. Transfusion-related sepsis due to *Serratia liquefaciens* in the United States. Transfusion 2000;40:931-5.

> Summary of 5 episodes of transfusion related sepsis and endotoxic shock due to *Serratia liquefaciens* in 5 whole blood donations. In the first case, a return of a 27-day-old hemolysed untransfused RBC led to a lookback of the random platelet from this donation, which showed that the platelet had been associated with the septic death of the recipient due to *Serratia liquefaciens*. Case 5 (an addendum) described a 26-day-old RBC that resulted in endotoxic shock of the recipient. Investigation of the platelet component revealed that the recipient had subsequently developed *Serratia liquefaciens* bacteremia. These two cases provide a good illustration that the contamination of platelet units result in sepsis or death can go unnoticed.

Skin preparation

Goldman M, Roy G, Frechette N, Decary F, Massicotte L, Delage G. Evaluation of donor skin disinfection methods. Transfusion 1997;37:309-12.

> Contact plates were used for antecubital skin cultures before and after skin disinfection of the antecubital fossa. Disinfection with povidone-iodine, isopropyl alcohol/iodine tinture, chlorhexidine gluconate/isopropyl alcohol and green-soap sponge/isopropyl alcohol were compared. Compared to the standard povidone-iodine method, isopropyl alcohol and tincture of iodine resulted in significantly less bacterial growth ($p < 0.001$). In this study, 13 of 30 subjects had more bacteria colonies present after skin disinfection with green soap and isopropyl alcohol than before disinfection!

McDonald CP, Lowe P, Roy A, Robbins S, Hartley S, Harrison JF, Slopecki A, Verlander N, Barbara JA. Evaluation of donor arm disinfection techniques. Vox Sang 2001 Apr;80(3):135-41.

> A direct swabbing and plating technique was used to enumerate bacteria present on the arm pre- and post-disinfection. Twelve donor arm disinfection techniques were evaluated. The Medi-Flex Adapted method, consisting of a 2-stage process with an initial application of isopropyl alcohol followed by tincture of iodine, produced the best arm disinfection. A percentage reduction in bacterial counts of 99.79% (logarithmic reduction of 2.67) was obtained. Post-disinfection, 70% of donors had bacterial counts of zero, and 98% had counts of 10 or less.

Diversion

De Korte D, Marcelis JH, Verhoeven AJ, Soeterboek AM. Diversion of first blood volume results in a reduction of bacterial contamination for whole-blood collections. Vox Sang. 2002 Jul;83(1):13-6.

A study from the Netherlands that showed that removal of the first 10 mL of donor blood was associated with a significant decrease in bacterial contamination (n=18,257 collections with 0.35% contamination compared with n=7,087 collections with a contamination rate of 0.21%, $p<0.05$) after diversion. It was concluded that the rate of bacterial contaminants in whole blood units could be reduced by diversion of the first 8-10 mL of collected volume, especially with respect to staphylococcal skin flora.

Bruneau C, Perez P, Chassaigne M, Allouch P, Audurier A, Gulian C, Janus G, Boulard G, De Micco P, Salmi LR, Noel L. Efficacy of a new collection procedure for preventing bacterial contamination of whole-blood donations. Transfusion. 2001;41:74-81.

A French study that cultured the first and second 15 mL of blood collected from 3,385 donations. While contamination was found in 76 (2.2%) donations, only 21 of the 76 were culture-positive in the second 15 mL of the collection. Diversion of the first 15 mL of the collection would have prevented the introduction of bacteria in 55 donations. It was concluded that excluding the first 15 mL of blood may reduce the rate of bacterial contamination in donations.

Growth and implications for the timing of sampling

Brecher ME, Holland PV, Pineda A, Tegtmeier G, Yomtovian R. Bacterial growth in inoculated platelets: Implications for bacterial detection and the extension of platelet storage. Transfusion 2000;40:1308-12.

The bacterial growth characteristics of 165 platelet units, each inoculated on the day of collection with one of the following organisms: *Bacillus cereus*, *Pseudomonas aeruginosa*, *Klebsiella pneumoniae*, *Serratia marcescens*, *Staphylococcus aureus* and *Staphylococcus epidermidis* (figure 4) has been published. All examples of *Bacillus cereus*, *Pseudomonas aeruginosa*, *Klebsiella pneumoniae*, *Serratia marcescens*, and *Staphylococcus aureus* had concentrations $\geq 10^2$ CFU/mL by day 3 following inoculation. By day 4 all units with these organisms contained $\geq 10^5$ CFU/mL. Units contaminated with *Staphylococcus epidermidis* showed slower and more varied growth. This study suggests that an assay capable of detecting 10^2 CFU/mL on day 3, or 10 CFU/mL on day 2 of storage, would detect the vast majority of bacterially contaminated platelet units. This paper also shows that with a variety of organisms, plateau growth is typically achieved by day 3 or 4 of storage.

Detection methodology

Staining

Barrett BB, Andersen JW, Anderson KC: Strategies for the avoidance of bacterial contamination of blood components. Transfusion 1993;33:228-33.

A study of 5,334 platelet units in which 8 yielded positive Gram stain results, 6 of which were negative by culture.

Nucleotide detection

Brecher ME, Hogan JJ, Boothe G, Kerr A, McClannan L, Jacobs MR, Yomtovian R, Chongokolwatana V, Tegtmeier G, Henderson S, Pineda A, Halling V, Kemper M, Kuramato K, Holland PV, Longiaru M. Platelet Bacterial Contamination and the Use of a Chemiluminescence Linked Universal Bacterial Ribosomal RNA Gene Probe. Transfusion, 1994;34:750-55.

A multicenter trial describing the use of a non-amplified chemiluminescence-linked universal bacterial rRNA probe confirmed the effectiveness of this technique in detecting platelet samples contaminated with one of four bacterial species. All platelet samples with bacterial concentrations of 2.1 x 10^5 CFU/mL or greater yielded positive results. In the range of 10^4 to 10^5 CFU/mL, 92% of *S. epidermidis* contaminated units were detected. In some cases, *S. aureus* was detected at levels as low as 10^2 to 10^3 CFU/mL.

Multi-reagent strips and swirling

Wagner SJ, Robinette D. Evaluation of swirling, pH, and glucose tests for the detection of bacterial contamination in platelet concentrates. Transfusion 1996;36:989-93.

This paper assessed pH and glucose by the use of reagent strips and swirling in platelet concentrates which had been inoculated with one of seven strains of bacteria. Overall, glucose concentrations, pH, and swirling became abnormal when the concentrations of bacteria reached 10^7 to 10^8 CFU/mL.

Burstain JM, Brecher ME, Workman K, et al. Rapid identification of bacterially contaminated platelets using reagent strips: glucose, and pH analysis as markers of bacterial metabolism. Transfusion 1997;37:255-58.

This paper evaluated the use of pH and glucose reagents in detecting contamination in platelets inoculated with five bacterial species. These investigators detected all bacteria at concentrations of greater than or equal to 10^7 CFU/mL and in some cases of *Staphylococcus aureus* and *Klebsiella pneumoniae* at levels of 10^3 to 10^5 CFU/mL. Overall, the sensitivity was 95% with a specificity of 98 to 100% at 10^7 CFU/mL.

Werch JB, Mhawech P, Stager CE, Banez EI, Lichtiger B. Detecting bacteria in platelet concentrates by use of reagent strips. Transfusion 2002;42:1027-31.

Prospective surveillance of 3,093 platelet concentrates at the MD Anderson Cancer Center in Houston, Texas, with reagent strips found 30 platelet concentrates with a glucose concentration or pH outside of their reference range. Two of the these platelets were found to be culture-positive for *Bacillus cereus*. Screening PC units by the reagent strip method resulted in 9.7 units per 1,000 being wasted, but prevented two patients from receiving a PC unit containing *B. cereus*.

Culture

Brecher ME, Means N, Jere CS, Heath D, Rothenberg S, Stutzman LC. Evaluation of the BacT/ALERT 3D® Microbial Detection System for platelet bacterial contamination: An analysis of 15 contaminating organisms. Transfusion 2001;41;477-82.

> Isolates of 15 organisms were inoculated into day-2 apheresis platelet units in order to obtain a final concentration of approximately 10 and 100 CFU/mL (2 units per organism) and cultured in replicate with the BacTAlert automated liquid culture system. With the exception of *P. acnes* (which is of questionable clinical significance), all of the contaminants were detected on average in < 25.6 hours.

Brecher ME, Heath D, Hay S, Rothenberg S, Stutzman LC. Evaluation of a new generation culture bottle using the BacT/ALERT 3D® Microbial Detection System on 9 common contaminating organisms found in platelet components. Transfusion 2002;42:774-9.

> Isolates of 9 organisms were inoculated into day-2 apheresis platelet units in order to obtain a final concentration of approximately 10 and 100 CFU/mL (2 units per organism) cultured in replicate with the BacTAlert automated liquid culture system and new generation culture bottles was compared to the current generation of bottles. Standard aerobic and anaerobic bottles were comparable.

Filtration

Buchholz DH, AuBuchon JP, Snyder EL, Kandler R, Piscitelli V, Pickard C, Napychank P, Edberg S. Effects of white cell reduction on the resistance of blood components to bacterial multiplication. Transfusion 1994;34:852-7.

> Two unit pools of whole blood were inoculated with 17 different organism (24 isolates) to approximately 1 CFU/ml (at 2 laboratories). The pools were split and processed into leukocyte-reduced (by filtration) or not-leukocyte-reduced red cell, plasma and platelet concentrates. Minimal to no growth was seen in 14 of the platelet pairs. In 4 pairs growth did not seem to be significantly affected by filtration and in 6 cases the WBC-reduction process lessened bacterial proliferation during 22· C storage compared to the paired unit that had not been WBC-reduced.

Holden F, Foley M, Devin G, Kinsella A, Murphy WG. Coagulase-negative staphylococcal contamination of whole blood and its components: The effects of WBC reduction. Transfusion 2000;40:1508-13.

> Whole blood units were inoculated with 19 different coagulase-negative *Staphylococcus* (CNS) isolates at 1-10 and 10-100 CFUs/mL. After an overnight hold at 22· C, the units were processed into components. For platelet concentrates, 6 (32%) of 19 grew bacteria before filtration and 1 of 18 after filtration (difference not statistically significant).

Wenz B, Ciavarella D, Freundlich L. Effect of prestorage white cell reduction on bacterial growth in platelet concentrates. Transfusion 1993;33:520-3.

Units of whole blood were inoculated with 1 of 5 species of bacterium at either 10 or 50 CFU/mL and then processed into platelet concentrates. *Klebsiella pneumoniae* failed to grow. With *Staphylococcus epidermidis*, *S. Aureus*, *Enterococcus faecalis*, and *Salmonella enteritidis*, although the concentration of bacteria immediately after inoculation was lower in the units reduced in white cells by filtration, no significant differences were observed thereafter.

Inactivation

Huston BM, Brecher ME, Bandarenko N. Lack of efficacy for conventional gamma irradiation of platelet concentrates to abrogate bacterial growth. Amer J Clin Path 1998;109:743-7.

This paper showed that exposure of *S. marcescen - or Staphyulococcus aureus-*contaminated platelet concentrates to gamma irradiation up to 75 Gy (3 times the normal amount of irradiation used with blood products) did not result in sterile platelet concentrates.

Lin L, Cook DN, Wiesehahn GP, et al. Photochemical inactivation of viruses and bacteria in platelet concentrates by use of a novel psoralen and long-wavelength ultraviolet light. Transfusion 1997;37:423-35.

Photochemical treatment with a novel psoralen, S-59 and UVA resulted in the $>10^{5.6}$ reduction in CFU of *Staphylococcus epidermidis* and $>10^{5.6}$ CFU of *Klebsiella pneumonieae* in platelet concentrates.

Knutson F, Alfonso R, Dupuis K, et al. Photochemical inactivation of bacteria and HIV in buffy-coat-derived platelet concentrates under conditions that preserve in vitro platelet function. Vox Sanguinis 2000; 78(4):209-16.

Buffy coat platelets photochemically treated with the psoralen S-59 and UV irradiation showed no growth with *Stapylococcus epidermidis, Staphylococcus aureus, Enterococcus faecalis, Enterobacter aerogenes, Pseudomonas aeruginosa, Serratia marcescens*, and *Klebsiella pneumoniae*. However, 1 of 2 platelets inoculated with *Bacillus cereus* grew similar to untreated control platelets. It was suspected that organisms capable of forming spores (such as *Bacillus*) may be resistant to photochemical inactivation.

Culture and Storage of Platelets for 7 Days

AuBuchon JP, Cooper LK, Leach MF, Zuaro DE, Schwartzman JD. Experience with universal bacterial culturing to detect contamination of apheresis platelet units in a hospital transfusion service. Transfusion 2002;42:855-61.

Using a sampling bag sterilely connected to 2,678 apheresis units cultured with the BacTAlert (standard aerobic bottle), 16 (0.6%) were positive on initial culture. Thirteen could be recultured, and all of these samples were negative. Shortly after the 2-year period of the study, 2 units (split from the same collection) were documented as growing coagulase-negative *Staphylococci* 12 hours after sampling. Units transfused on Day 6 or 7 (n = 40) yielded expected clinical responses, and CCI available on 21 recipients 10 to 60 minutes after transfusion demonstrated acceptable results (mean, 14,400 ± 8,800; median, 12,191; 90% > 7500). It was concluded that the cost of culturing could be mitigated with extension of the storage period, and clinical experience with units held for 6 or 7 days was satisfactory.

Dumont LJ, AuBuchon JP, Whitley P, Herschel LH, Johnson A, McNeil D, Sawyer S, Jill JC, Roger JC. Seven-day storage of single-donor platelets: recovery and survival in an autologous transfusion study. Transfusion 2002;42: 847-54.

> WBC-reduced, single-donor platelets (n = 24) were collected and stored by standard methods at two sites. In vitro platelet characteristics were adequately maintained over 7 days. Day 5 platelets had better radio labeled recovery (63.0 ± 4.36 vs. 53.9 ± 4.36%, p < 0.0001) and survival (161 ± 8.1 vs. 133 ± 8.1 hr, p = 0.006) than Day 7 platelets adjusting for radioisotope, center, and donor effects. However, the declines in recovery and survival noted were less than used previously to gain licensure of 7-day storage and were felt to be unlikely to be clinically significant. The authors concluded that extension of storage to 7 days could be implemented with bacterial screening methods to select out contaminated components without a significant effect on the platelet efficacy compared to 5-day components.

Abstracts:

In addition to the above referenced papers, there are several possible or promising methodologies that have as yet been described only in abstract form. These include, but are not limited to:

The Pall bacterial detection system (BDS) system

McDonald CP, Smith R, Colvin R, Roy A, Wall C, Hartley S, Barbara JAT. Study to determine the sensitivity of the Pall bacterial detection system. Vox Sang 2002;83 Supplement 2 Abstract 015.

McDonald CP, Smith R, Colvin R, Roy A, Wall C, Hartley S, Robbins S, Barbara JAT. Evaluation of the Pall bacterial detection system (BDS). Vox Sang 2002;83 Supplement 2 Abstract 018.

The Gambro riboflavin pathogen reduction system

Palavecino EL, Jacobs MR, Goodrich RP, McBurney LL, Goodrich TB, Yomtovian RA. Photochemical decontamination of bacteria: Analysis of log and stationary growth phases.

Transfusion 2001;41 Supplement 88S-89S.

Appendix 2. Association Bulletin #03-7

ASSOCIATION BULLETIN

#03-07

Date: May 16, 2003

To: AABB Members

From: Roger Dodd, PhD - President
Karen Shoos Lipton, JD - Chief Executive Officer

Re: Guidance on Implementation of New Bacteria Reduction and Detection Standard

On March 3, 2003, the AABB Blood Bank/Transfusion Service Standards Program Unit, with the approval of the AABB Board of Directors, issued the following new standard for inclusion in the 22nd edition of *Standards for Blood Banks and Transfusion Services,* scheduled for implementation on November 1, 2003:

5.1.5.1 The blood bank or transfusion service shall have methods to limit and detect bacterial contamination in all platelet components. Standard 5.6.2 applies.

5.1.5.1.1 Standard 5.1.5.1 shall be implemented by March 1, 2004.

Standard 5.6.2, which is referenced in 5.1.5.1, reads as follows:

5.6.2 The venipuncture site shall be prepared so as to minimize the risk of bacterial contamination. Green soap shall not be used.

The purpose of this Association Bulletin is to provide guidance to the membership in developing strategies to implement this new standard and to supplement the information provided in Association Bulletin 02-08.

While bacterial contamination of platelets has long been recognized as the most common infectious risk of transfusion therapy,[1-3] there is no single defined strategy, available at this time, to prevent platelet bacterial contamination. However, a combination of strategies aimed simultaneously at limiting entry of bacteria into platelet units and at detecting bacteria gaining entry into platelet units can act in synergy to greatly reduce the risk of platelet bacterial contamination.

Phlebotomy-related bacterial contamination is reduced through the use of apheresis platelets wit the associated single phlebotomy. Pooled whole-blood-derived platelets are associated with phlebotomies from multiple donors.[4-5] However, the applications of this strategy are limited given the significant role of whole blood derived platelets in transfusion medicine and due to the insufficient amount of apheresis platelets to meet clinical needs on a national level.

Methods to Limit Bacterial Contamination of Platelet Units

Because the most frequent source of platelet bacterial contamination is associated with phlebotomy, it is vital that strategies be implemented to limit phlebotomy associated bacterial contamination. Of the currently available strategies to limit bacterial contamination of platelet units, the following will meet the requirements of standard 5.1.5.1:

- Careful Phlebotomy Technique – The 22nd edition of AABB *Standards for Blood Banks and Transfusion Services*, Standard 5.6.2, contains new requirements for arm preparation. In addition, use of an iodine-based scrub is correlated with improved bacterial disinfection.[6] An arm preparation of alcohol and chlorhexidine is recommended for donors with an allergy to iodine. Venipuncture sites should be selected to avoid areas of scarring or dimpling. Scarred skin harbors an increased quantity of bacteria.[7]
- Phlebotomy Diversion – Diversion of the initial 20-30 mL of the blood collection so that it does not enter the collection container has been shown to reduce the quantity of bacteria associated with the phlebotomy process. Diversion is particularly effective in reducing contamination associated with coagulase-negative *Staphylococcus*, the most common organism implicated in platelet bacterial contamination.[8] The use of diversion pouches is particularly important for facilities that prepare whole blood derived platelets. In the absence of an entirely apheresis-based platelet supply, the use of diversion pouches is a necessary element of satisfying the requirement to limit bacteria in platelet components. Several blood bag manufacturers have developed collection sets incorporating a diversion pouch. The blood collected into the diversion pouch is used for viral marker testing. While the availability of diversion methods can be used as a criterion for vendor qualification when contracting for purchase of blood collection bags, the AABB is not recommending that blood collection facilities attempt to change their blood bag suppliers in haste, or without due consideration for all the logistical issues such a change might entail. The current expectation is that diversion methods will be made available by all collection bag suppliers for their specific bags. Although not addressed in *Standards for Blood Banks and Transfusion Services,* collection facilities are encouraged to consider the impact of diversion strategies on other products that are susceptible to bacterial contamination.
- Use of Apheresis Platelets: Phlebotomy-related bacterial contamination is reduced through the use of apheresis platelets with the associated single phlebotomy.

The nature of the requirement to "limit" bacterial contamination also depends on the activities performed within the facility. The strategies discussed above are primarily performed immediately prior to and during collection. A hospital that does not collect platelet components will have met this requirement if the supplier meets it.

Methods to Detect Bacterial Contamination of Platelet Units

Several strategies that differ in sensitivity and specificity are currently available to detect platelet bacterial contamination and will fulfill the requirements of Standard 5.1.5.1. In selecting a detection system, the facility should consider the sensitivity of the method for preventing clinically significant contamination together with the timing of the proposed application. Less sensitive methods should be used as close as possible to the time of issue.

While all processes and procedures must be validated in accordance with *Standards*, the extent of validation is largely a function of the risk associated with a given methodology. Methods approved by the Food and Drug Administration (FDA) require less extensive validation than use of dipstick or staining techniques.

Bacteria Detection strategies include:

- Culture Methods
  Use of a culture method for detection of platelet bacterial contamination currently achieves the best combination of test sensitivity and specificity, detecting as few as 1 bacterial organism per mL (1 CFU/mL) of platelet sample. In order to achieve this sensitivity, however, platelet units must be held for a minimum of 24 hours prior to the time of sampling (to allow bacteria to grow to levels sufficient to ensure that any existing bacteria will appear in a sample) and must be incubated for a minimum of 24 additional hours to grow bacteria to detectable levels. [9-11] This is the optimal detection method, at this time, for testing apheresis platelets.

  Two culture methods, the BacT/ALERT (bioMerieux, Inc., Durham, NC) and Pall Bacteria Detection System (BDS) (Medsep Corp, Covina, CA), have been cleared by the FDA for quality control (QC) monitoring of leukocyte-reduced apheresis platelets. The BDS is also approved for use with leukocyte-reduced whole blood derived platelets. Information about the use of these methods is contained in the package inserts for both devices (Information for Use).

  Either method can be implemented in the blood collecting or transfusing facility. While both techniques are considered to be culture methods, the BDS is designed to read the percentage of oxygen in the sample (as a marker for bacterial growth) in a sample pouch at a single time-point, generally close in proximity to the time of transfusion. In contrast, the BacT/ALERT (or similar system) provides continuous monitoring of carbon dioxide production (a marker for bacterial growth) for the duration of platelet storage. It is estimated that at least 90% of bacterially contaminated platelets will be positive by BacT/ALERT prior to transfusion. [10] Because the manufacturer recommends that monitoring continue until platelet unit outdate, there may be cases in which bacterially contaminated platelets can be identified only following transfusion.

  Other culture methods such as the BACTEC system (Becton Dickinson, Franklin Lanes, NJ) that employ a method that is comparable to the BacT/ALERT, or a manual culture plate method may also be used to meet standard 5.1.5.1. However, in the absence of specific FDA clearance of this or any other method mentioned below for monitoring platelet QC, these methods would need to be validated by the end user for efficacy in detecting bacteria. Given the complexities of these issues, transfusion facilities are encouraged to initiate a discussion and coordinate plans for platelet bacteria detection strategies with their blood provider prior to selecting a detection method.

  Facilities are reminded that QC monitoring of bacteria detection may not be used for product labeling even if an FDA-cleared method is used. In addition, facilities should consider the need to identify the microbiological isolate and to address product management/quarantine/discard and appropriate donor and patient follow-up related to positive cultures. Transfusion facilities are encouraged to discuss these questions with their blood providers and begin developing appropriate policies, processes and procedures to define the appropriate actions to be taken in response to such events. Further AABB guidance will be forthcoming.
- Staining Methods
  Gram's stain, acridine orange stain or Wright's stain have been used to detect bacterial organisms in platelet units. These methods are less sensitive than a culture method, estimated to detect at best from 10^4 CFU/mL organisms/CFU (for acridine orange) to approximately 10^5 CFU/mL – 10^6 CFU/mL (for Gram's and Wright's stain). Application of the staining methods, given their limited sensitivity, must be performed as close as possible to the time when a platelet unit is issued for transfusion so that the test result reflects the condition of the product at that time. If the test is performed earlier, a negative result would not be reflective of bacterial growth during storage. Despite the reduced

sensitivity of the staining methods, cases of bacterially contaminated platelet units have been successfully interdicted by application of the Gram's stain.[12]

- Dipstick
  Multireagent strips have been shown to detect the vast majority of bacterially contaminated platelet units with bacteria levels $>10^7$ CFU/mL and in some cases to level of 10^3 CFU/mL.[13, 14, 15] Use of multireagent strips has been validated in the literature with Baxter PL732 CPD bags and with Medsep CLX CP2D bags. A glucose level of <250 mg/dL in the PL732 CPD bags, ≤500 mg/dL in the CLX CP2D bags or a pH of <7.0 were predictive of bacterial contamination. In other test systems, validation of normal ranges will be required. In one small study of Fenwal CS3000 apheresis platelets, glucose was frequently reduced to such a low level on storage day 5 as to preclude the usefulness of the glucose determination. As with staining, this procedure must be performed as close i time as possible to the issuance of a platelet unit.
- Swirling
  Normally functioning platelets have a discoid morphology. In fresh platelets, about 60% c platelets are discs and the remainder become spheres. When the platelet container is gently rotated and viewed through a light source, these discoid platelets exhibit a shimmering or swirling phenomenon due to their alignment with flow, as illustrated below When platelets are subject to metabolic disturbances such as those associated with cold storage temperatures, prolonged in-vitro storage and low pH they become spherical and lose their ability to exhibit in-vitro swirling. This method, advocated in the past as a surrogate detection strategy for bacterial contamination, is difficult to implement reliably, as interpretation of the research is highly subjective[16], difficult to validate and limited in sensitivity to bacterial levels of generally $> 10^7$ CFU/mL. Nonetheless, it may be successful in identifying and interdicting platelet units contaminated with large quantities of bacteria[15] when applied immediately prior to issue of the platelet unit for transfusion.

While swirling may be an effective supplemental technique, it does not independently constitute a method to detect bacteria as required by the standard. Swirling does, however, meet the requirement of Standard 5.17, "Final Inspection of Blood and Components Before Issue," which requires that blood and components be inspected at the time of issue. Facilities that currently use this technique to meet Standard 5.17 are encouraged to continue doing so.

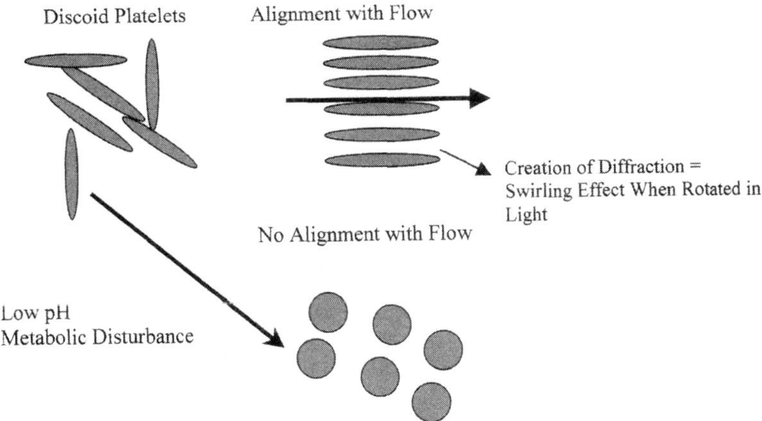

Conclusions

Given the important role of whole-blood-derived platelets in transfusion therapy, it may not be possible to substitute apheresis platelets for whole-blood-derived platelets. Careful attention to phlebotomy technique and selection of a phlebotomy bag vendor employing phlebotomy diversion should reduce the level and extent of contamination of pooled platelet units.

Selection of a detection strategy is far more complex. There is, at the present time, no method cleared by the FDA that may be cited in product labeling. While the FDA has cleared two culture methods--the BacT/ALERT and BDS culture systems--as QC monitoring methods for platelet bacterial contamination, the package inserts limit application of these methods to leukocyte-reduced apheresis units, in the case of BacT/ALERT, and leukocyte-reduced apheresis and whole-blood-derived platelets in the case of BDS. In addition, both methods reduce useable platelet shelf life significantly because of the mandatory storage hold time prior to culture and incubation time during culture.

Another logical approach would be application of a sensitive culture detection strategy to the actual pool of platelets. However, this approach is limited by the current FDA-required expiration time of 4 hours following pooling. The FDA has already been approached about the need to extend the expiration time for pooled platelets and has discussed data that could be used to allow for a change in this requirement at a recent meeting of its Blood Products Advisory Committee.

The standard may be implemented by the blood provider, the transfusion facility or a combination of both. Those steps performed by a blood provider in fulfillment of this standard do not need to be duplicated by the transfusion facility. Due to the complex issues surrounding responsibility for performing bacteria detection, more detailed information will be forthcoming.

It is apparent, in the near term, that hospitals and blood providers will need to work closely together to develop complementary and cost-effective strategies to conform to standard 5.1.5.1. As an example, should the blood provider elect to test only apheresis platelet inventory with one of the FDA-cleared culture methods, the transfusing facility will need to select a supplemental detection method for their whole-blood-derived platelets.

Facilities are encouraged to initiate implementation of this standard by beginning a dialogue with the blood provider or hospital customer to identify a likely strategy for addressing the new AABB standard (including the expected time frame for implementation and added product costs); and to plan a testing strategy for whole- blood-derived platelets and apheresis platelets collected on-site

Because this is a rapidly evolving area, the ultimate approach to interdicting platelet bacterial contamination is not yet clearly defined. The AABB is committed to providing ongoing leadership to help with the successful implementation of this standard, assessing new strategies and technologies, and providing the necessary guidance as they become available.

References

1. Blajchman MA. Incidence and significance of the bacterial contamination contamination of blood components. Dev Biol (Basel) 2002;108:59-67.
2. Jacobs MR, Palavecino E, Yomtovian R. Don't bug me: The problem of bacterial contamination of blood components--challenges and solutions. Transfusion 2001; 41:1131-4.
3. Goodnough LT, Shander A, Brecher ME. Transfusion medicine: Looking to the future. Lancet 2003;361:161-9.
4. Dykstra A, Jacobs M, Yomtovian R. Prospective microbiologic surveillance (PMS) of random donor (RDP) and single donor apheresis platelets (SDP). (abstract) Transfusion 1998;38 (suppl):104S.
5. Ness P, Braine H, King K, et al. Single-donor platelets reduce the risk of septic platelet transfusion reactions. Transfusion 2001;41:857-61.
6. Goldman M, Roy G, Frechette N, et al. Evaluation of donor skin disinfection methods. Transfusion 1997;37:309-12.
7. Anderson KC, Lew MA, Gorgone BC, et al. Transfusion-related sepsis after prolonged platelet storage. Am J Med 1986;81:405-11.
8. De Korte D, Marcelis JH, Verhoeven AJ , Soeterboek AM. Diversion of first blood volume results in a reduction of bacterial contamination for whole blood collections. Vox Sang 2002;83:13-16.
9. McDonald CP, Roy A, Lowe P, et al.Evaluation of the BacT/ALERT automated blood culture system for detecting bacteria and measuring their growth kinetics in leucodepleted and non-leucodepleted platelet concentrates. Vox Sang 2001;81:154-60.
10. Brecher ME, Means N, Jere CS, et al. Evaluation of an automated culture system for detecting bacterial contamination of platelets: An analysis with 15 contaminating organisms. Transfusion 2001;41:477-82.
11. AuBuchon JP, Cooper LK, Leach MF, et al. Experience with universal bacterial culturing to detect contamination of apheresis platelet units in a hospital transfusion service. Transfusion 2002;42:855-61.
12. Yomtovian R, Lazarus HM, Goodnough LT, et al. A prospective microbiologic surveillance program to detect and prevent transfusion of bacterially contaminated platelets. Transfusion 1993;33:902-9.
13. Burstain JM, Brecher ME, Workman K, et al. Rapid identification of bacterially contaminated platelets using reagent strips: Glucose and pH analysis as markers of bacterial metabolism. Transfusion 1997;37:255-8.
14. Werch JB, Mhawech P, Stager CE, et al. Detecting bacteria in platelet concentrates by use of reagent strips. Transfusion 2002;42:1027-31.

15. Wagner SJ, Robinette D. Evaluation of swirling, pH, and glucose tests for the detection o bacterial contamination in platelet concentrates. Transfusion 1996;36:989-93.
16. Bertolini F, Murphy S. A multicenter inspection of the swirling phenomenon in platelet concentrates prepared in routine practice. Biomedical Excellence for Safer Transfusion (BEST) Working Party of the International Society of Blood Transfusion. Transfusion 1996;36:128-32.

Appendix 3. President's Message*

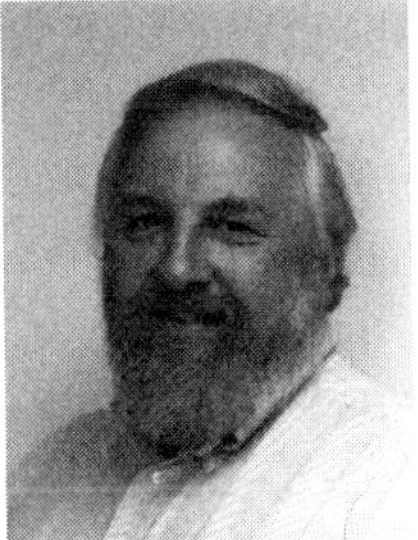

Roger Y. Dodd, PhD

Our Voice at Work

In March 2003, AABB's Board of Directors approved the 22nd edition of *Standards for Blood Banks and Transfusion Services*. Over the years, the standards have introduced many required activities—some more welcome than others—but all aimed at improving transfusion safety for patients. As a board and as an organization, we have received extensive feedback about many of these initiatives from you, the members. In the past couple of years, the most common lament has been the inability of the blood banking community to prioritize, by importance, threats to transfusion safety.

The new edition of *Standards* presents the transfusion and blood banking community with a unique opportunity, that of responding to an issue identified as one of the greatest threats to transfusion safety. Unlike other challenges, the threat of bacterial contamination has been an issue owned and highlighted by our own membership.

One year ago, the AABB Board asked two prestigious committees, the Transfusion Transmitted Diseases Committee and

*From *AABB News*, May/June, 2003

the Clinical Transfusion Medicine Committee, to assess current risks to the blood supply. Members of these committees, experts in blood banking and transfusion medicine from all sectors of our profession, concluded that the No. 1 risk to infection-related transfusion recipients is bacterial contamination.

Since that time, the consensus of the blood community over the need to address bacterial contamination has been growing. In 2003, members of our own medical discipline wrote an open letter to the blood community, urging them to address the risk in a meaningful way. In January, the Advisory Committee on Blood Safety and Availability adopted a resolution, calling on the federal government to take action to detect bacterial contamination in blood components. The College of American Pathologists recently incorporated a requirement in its Transfusion Medicine Checklist, requiring that laboratories have a system to detect the presence of bacteria in Platelet components.

Unlike during other threats to blood safety, existing or theoretical, that have been hyped by the media and the public, the groundswell for reducing bacterial contamination has come from the blood banking and transfusion medicine community. The Standards Committee listened to our profession and took action.

Unfortunately, the solution to the problem will prove to be as difficult—if not more so—than identifying the problem. There is no clear path to eliminating the risk; there is no unanimity about how the standard should be written to effect the change. There are regulatory hurdles to be addressed if the solutions are to be effective, and there are unbudgeted costs associated with the fix. But these obstacles are ours to address, without the constraints of regulatory timelines and public pressure to act.

Our most commonly voiced complaint today is that we are forced to operate under an agenda that we do not control. Bacterial detection presents us with an opportunity to control our own destiny, to demonstrate that we can and do lead the profession, and that our paramount concern is to improve transfusion safety for patients. It is an opportunity that we cannot allow to pass.

Index

Page numbers in italics represent tables

Q-R

U-V

W

Y